Chia Seeds for IBS

Managing Constipation and Digestive Issues

Alice Klayn

Disclaimer

The information provided in ***Chia Seeds for IBS: Managing Constipation and Digestive Issues**"* by **Alice Klayn** is intended for educational and informational purposes only.

While the content is based on thorough research and the author's expertise in nutrition and digestive health. Always seek the advice of your physician or other qualified health provider with any questions you may have regarding a medical condition or dietary changes.

The author and publisher disclaim any liability for any adverse effects or consequences resulting from the use or application of any information, suggestions, or recommendations in this book. Individual results may vary, and the efficacy of chia seeds and dietary changes can differ based on personal health conditions and responses.

Introduction

Welcome to ***"Chia Seeds for IBS: Managing Constipation and Digestive Issues"*** If you're one of the millions struggling with Irritable Bowel Syndrome (IBS), you know all too well how it can disrupt your daily life. The discomfort, the unpredictability, and the constant search for relief can feel overwhelming. But what if a tiny seed could help you regain control over your digestive health?

Enter chia seeds—the nutrient powerhouse that's quickly becoming a game-changer for those battling IBS. Packed with fiber, omega-3 fatty acids, and antioxidants, these tiny wonders not only enhance your meals but also offer remarkable benefits for gut health.

In this ebook, we'll explore how incorporating chia seeds into your diet can help alleviate constipation and other digestive issues, empowering you to reclaim your comfort and confidence.

We'll delve into the science behind chia seeds and their ability to support digestive function, providing you with actionable tips on how to seamlessly integrate them into your daily routine.

From simple recipes to creative ideas for incorporating chia seeds into your favorite dishes, this guide will equip you with everything you need to start your journey toward better digestive health.

So, whether you're seeking natural remedies or simply looking for ways to make your meals more enjoyable, you've come to the right place

Chapter 1: Understanding IBS and Constipation

Characterized by chronic abdominal pain, bloating, and changes in bowel habits, IBS presents a complex condition that can significantly affect an individual's quality of life. While it does not cause permanent damage to the intestines, its symptoms can be distressing and confusing.

The exact etiology of IBS remains an ongoing topic of research. It is important to note that IBS is a functional gastrointestinal disorder, meaning it is diagnosed based on a group of symptoms rather than a specific identifiable organic cause. The diagnosis is primarily made using the Rome criteria, which classify IBS into several subtypes according to the predominant bowel habit: IBS with diarrhea (IBS-D), IBS with constipation (IBS-C), mixed IBS (IBS-M), and IBS without subtype.

Symptoms of IBS

The characteristic symptoms of IBS include:

Abdominal Pain: Usually relieved by bowel movements and can vary in intensity and location.

Bloating and Distension: Many people report feeling a sense of fullness or bloating in the abdomen.

Altered Bowel Habits: Depending on the subtype of IBS, individuals may experience diarrhea, constipation, or a combination of both. In IBS-C, the predominant symptom is constipation, which can further complicate the condition and lead to increased discomfort.

IBS and Constipation

Constipation is one of the most troublesome components of IBS. Defined as having fewer than three bowel movements per week, constipation can manifest in various ways, including difficulty passing stools, the sensation of incomplete evacuation, and hard or lumpy stools. Many individuals with IBS-C may also experience infrequent bowel movements along with abdominal pain and discomfort.

The interaction between IBS and constipation is complex. The intestinal dysfunction observed in IBS is influenced by several factors, including:

Intestinal Motility: In IBS-C, the speed at which food moves through the digestive tract is slower than normal, leading to the buildup of stool in the intestines.

Visceral Hypersensitivity: Many individuals with IBS have an exaggerated response to normal intestinal distension. This hypersensitivity can lead to increased abdominal pain and discomfort, contributing to the perception of constipation.

Psychological Factors: Stress, anxiety, and depression have been linked to IBS symptoms. Psychological factors can exacerbate digestive issues and trigger bowel irregularities.

Dietary Influences: Certain foods and eating patterns can cause symptoms. For example, diets high in refined carbohydrates and sugars and low in fiber may contribute to constipation.

Diagnosis of IBS-C

Diagnosing IBS, particularly IBS-C, often involves a combination of medical history, symptom evaluation, and exclusion of other gastrointestinal disorders. Some standard diagnostic tests include:

Blood Tests: To rule out infections, inflammation, or other underlying conditions.

Stool Tests: To check for signs of infection or malabsorption.

Colonoscopy: Especially in individuals over a certain age or with alarming symptoms, to visualize the colon and rule out organic diseases.

It's essential for those experiencing persistent gastrointestinal issues to seek medical advice to receive an accurate diagnosis and rule out other conditions.

Management of IBS and Constipation

Managing IBS and its symptoms, particularly constipation, often requires a multifaceted approach. Treatment strategies may include:

1. Dietary Modifications

Diet plays a critical role in managing IBS symptoms. Some recommendations include:

Increasing Fiber Intake: Gradually increasing both soluble and insoluble fiber can help regulate bowel movements. However, for some, high fiber may exacerbate symptoms, so it's crucial to tailor the approach to the individual.

Keeping a Food Diary: Tracking food intake and symptoms can help identify trigger foods and patterns.

Hydration: Adequate fluid intake is vital for promoting healthy digestion and preventing constipation.
2. Medications

Several medications can be prescribed to help manage IBS-C symptoms, including:

Laxatives: Over-the-counter options like osmotic laxatives can help soften stools and promote bowel movements.

Prescription Medications: Such as Linaclotide or Plecanatide, which stimulate bowel motility and reduce constipation.

3. Psychological Therapies

Cognitive Behavioral Therapy (CBT) and other psychological interventions can significantly improve symptoms. Mindfulness and stress management techniques also help in managing the psychological aspects of IBS.

4. Regular Physical Activity

Exercise can enhance gut motility and is an essential component of a healthy lifestyle, contributing to the overall well-being of individuals with IBS.

Irritable Bowel Syndrome, particularly the subtype characterized by constipation, is a multifaceted condition that requires a comprehensive understanding of its symptoms, triggers, and management strategies. By recognizing the complexities of IBS, individuals can navigate their condition more effectively, find relief from uncomfortable symptoms, and improve their quality of life.

Definition and Types of IBS (Irritable Bowel Syndrome)

This chapter aims to provide a comprehensive definition of IBS, explore its underlying characteristics, and categorize its various types. By delving into these aspects, we can develop a better understanding of this multifaceted condition and its implications on health and well-being.

Definition of IBS

Irritable Bowel Syndrome is defined as a functional gastrointestinal disorder characterized by chronic abdominal pain and discomfort, accompanied by alterations in bowel habits. These bowel habit changes may include episodes of diarrhea, constipation, or alternating between both. Importantly, IBS is classified as a "functional" disorder because it does not cause significant morphological changes in the gastrointestinal tract, which means that standard medical examinations (such as colonoscopy or imaging) typically reveal no structural abnormalities.

The symptoms experienced by individuals with IBS can vary widely in intensity and presentation. While the exact cause of IBS is still not well understood, it is believed to be related to a combination of factors, including diet, gut-brain interactions, hormonal changes, and gut microbiota abnormalities. The condition can affect individuals of any age, but it is more commonly diagnosed in younger adults and women.

Symptoms of IBS

The symptoms of IBS are generally categorized into two main groups: gastrointestinal (GI) symptoms and non-GI symptoms.

Gastrointestinal Symptoms:

Abdominal Pain and Cramping: This is a hallmark symptom that typically correlates with bowel movements. The pain may be relieved after defecation.

Bloating and Gas: Many individuals report a feeling of fullness or swelling in the abdomen, often accompanied by excessive gas.

Changes in Bowel Habits: These can manifest as diarrhea, constipation, or alternating between both. Each type of IBS is defined by the predominant bowel habit.

Non-Gastrointestinal Symptoms:

Fatigue: Individuals with IBS often report fatigue, which can be exacerbated by the stress of managing chronic symptoms.

Mental Health Issues: Increased levels of anxiety and depression have been observed in individuals with IBS, possibly due to the chronic nature of symptoms and the impact on daily life.

Sleep Disturbances: Many people with IBS experience difficulty sleeping, which can further compound fatigue and affect overall health.

Types of IBS

IBS is classified into four main types, primarily based on the predominant bowel habit experienced by the individual. Understanding these types can facilitate more effective treatment strategies tailored to individual needs.

1. IBS with Predominant Diarrhea (IBS-D)

Individuals with IBS-D predominantly experience frequent urges to have bowel movements accompanied by loose or watery stools. Symptoms often worsen after meals and can present with urgency, often leading to anxiety about accessing bathroom facilities.

2. IBS with Predominant Constipation (IBS-C)

IBS-C is characterized by infrequent bowel movements and straining during defecation, with patients often reporting hard or lumpy stools. Persistent abdominal pain and bloating accompany the constipation, leading to discomfort and dissatisfaction.

3. Mixed IBS (IBS-M)

In IBS-M, individuals experience alternating patterns of both diarrhea and constipation. This variability can lead to unpredictability in symptoms, further complicating the management of the condition. Patients may find that stress or certain foods can exacerbate their symptoms.

4. Unsubtyped IBS (IBS-U)

The term IBS-U is used for individuals who exhibit symptoms consistent with IBS but do not meet the specific criteria for any of the above subtypes. This category is more inclusive and recognizes that IBS can manifest in various ways that may not fit neatly into defined patterns.

Understanding the definition and types of Irritable Bowel

Syndrome is crucial for both patients and healthcare providers. Recognizing the different manifestations of IBS can lead to more effective diagnoses and individualized treatment plans.

Symptoms and Complications of IBS-Related Constipation

Among the subtypes of IBS, constipation-predominant IBS—often referred to as IBS-C—is particularly common. This chapter delves into the symptoms associated with IBS-C, outlines its complications, and highlights the importance of managing the condition effectively to improve patient quality of life.

Understanding IBS-Related Constipation

IBS-C affects millions of people worldwide, often leading to significant discomfort and disruption in daily activities. Unlike typical constipation, which can be defined by a strict number of bowel movements or stool consistency, IBS-C is characterized by a combination of symptoms that vary in intensity and presentation from one individual to another. These symptoms can lead to a profound impact on a person's physical and emotional well-being.

Common Symptoms

Abdominal Pain and Cramping:

Abdominal discomfort is a hallmark of IBS-C. Patients often describe the pain as cramp-like or bloating that is relieved after bowel movements. The intensity and location of the pain can vary, complicating diagnosis and management.

Infrequent Bowel Movements:

Affected individuals may experience fewer than three bowel movements per week. The stools are often hard, dry, or pellet-like in consistency, which can cause straining during passage.

Difficulty Passing Stools:

Many individuals with IBS-C report that while they feel the urge to defecate, they struggle to pass stool, leading to a sense of incomplete evacuation. This feeling can be frustrating and disheartening.

Bloating and Gas:

Bloating is a prevalent symptom reported by those with IBS-C. This sensation of fullness or swelling in the abdomen is frequently accompanied by increased gas, contributing to discomfort and a feeling of heaviness.

Change in Stool Appearance:

Individuals may notice changes in the form of their stool in addition to infrequency. Stools may vary from hard and lumpy to soft and even watery, depending on the dietary intake, stress levels, and other factors.

Nausea:

Some patients may experience nausea, particularly during active flare-ups. This symptom can contribute to decreased appetite and avoidance of certain foods.

Emotional and Psychological Symptoms

The impact of IBS-C is not limited to physical symptoms; it is often intertwined with emotional and psychological challenges. Many patients report feelings of anxiety, depression, and social withdrawal due to the unpredictability and discomfort associated with their gastrointestinal symptoms.

Complications of IBS-C

While IBS-C is generally considered a benign condition, it can lead to complications that may significantly affect an individual's quality of life and overall health.

Quality of Life Impairment:

The chronic nature of IBS-C can lead to considerable impairment in quality of life. Patients may limit their social interactions or avoid specific situations (like traveling) for fear of not having access to a restroom or experiencing an episode.

Impact on Nutrition:

Individuals may resort to restrictive diets in an attempt to manage their symptoms, potentially leading to nutritional deficiencies. Some may eliminate foods that are important sources of fiber and nutrients out of fear that they will exacerbate constipation or cause discomfort.

Chronic Pain and Discomfort:

Persistent abdominal pain can lead to a chronic pain cycle, which may require medical intervention and ongoing monitoring. The consistent discomfort can also increase one's reliance on pain medication, which may introduce further complications.

Co-existing Conditions:

Patients with IBS-C often present with other health concerns, such as fibromyalgia or mental health disorders like anxiety and depression. The interplay between these conditions can complicate treatment and management of IBS-C itself.

Delayed Diagnosis and Treatment:

Symptoms of IBS-C can mimic other gastrointestinal disorders, such as inflammatory bowel disease (IBD) or colorectal cancer. This overlap can lead to delays in diagnosis and treatment, potentially contributing to increased anxiety and fear among patients.

Medication Side Effects:

The pursuit of relief through pharmacological means can lead to adverse effects. Laxatives, often used as a first-line therapy for constipation, can cause dependency and result in worsening symptoms if overused or misused.

Understanding the complexities of IBS-C is paramount in implementing effective treatment strategies that enhance patient outcomes and improve quality of life. Through heightened awareness and education, both patients and clinicians can work collaboratively towards managing this challenging condition.

Chapter 2: The Nutritional Powerhouse of Chia Seeds

Despite their small size, these tiny white or black seeds pack a big punch and offer a wide variety of nutrients that have been celebrated by cultures around the world for centuries. From ancient Aztec warriors to modern health enthusiasts, chia seeds have earned their reputation as a nutritional powerhouse, making them a staple in health-conscious diets.

A Brief History

Chia seeds, derived from the plant *Salvia hispanica*, have a rich history that dates back to the ancient civilizations of Mesoamerica. The word "chia" comes from the Aztec word meaning "oily," and these seeds were highly valued for their nutritional properties and versatility. The Aztecs used chia seeds not only as a staple food source but also as a means of energy during long journeys and strenuous activities. For them, chia seeds were not just a food source; they symbolized strength and endurance.

Today, chia seeds have resurfaced as a staple in modern diets, recognized for their impressive nutritional profile and health benefits. This chapter will delve into the composition of chia seeds and explore what makes them such a remarkable addition to our diet.

A Nutritional Analysis

Chia seeds stand out for their impressive combination of macronutrients, vitamins, and minerals. Here's a closer look at their nutritional composition:

1. Omega-3 Fatty Acids

One of the most notable features of chia seeds is their high content of alpha-linolenic acid (ALA), a type of plant-based omega-3 fatty acid. Just two tablespoons (28 grams) of chia seeds provide approximately 5 grams of ALA, making them one of the richest sources of omega-3 found in plant foods. Omega-3s play a crucial role in heart health, as they help reduce inflammation, lower blood pressure, and potentially decrease the risk of heart disease.

2. Fiber Powerhouse

Chia seeds are an exceptional source of dietary fiber, containing about 11 to 12 grams per two-tablespoon serving. This high fiber content promotes digestive health, aiding in regularity and supporting gut health. Additionally, soluble fiber helps slow digestion and may stabilize blood sugar levels, contributing to a feeling of fullness that can assist with weight management.

3. Protein Punch

While they are not as protein-rich as some legumes or animal products, chia seeds still offer a significant amount of protein for a plant-based source. Two tablespoons provide approximately 4 grams of protein, including all nine essential amino acids. This makes chia seeds an excellent addition to vegetarian and vegan diets, as they provide a complete source of protein that is often lacking in plant-based foods.

4. Essential Minerals

Chia seeds are also a treasure trove of essential minerals, including calcium, magnesium, phosphorus, and iron. Calcium is vital for healthy bones, while magnesium plays a critical role in muscle function and energy production. The inclusion of iron is particularly beneficial for those following plant-based diets, as it helps prevent anemia and supports overall energy levels.

5. Antioxidant Properties

Beyond their macronutrient and micronutrient profile, chia seeds are rich in antioxidants. These powerful compounds combat oxidative stress in the body by neutralizing free radicals, which can cause cellular damage. The antioxidant content in chia seeds contributes to overall health and may reduce the risk of chronic diseases.

How to Incorporate Chia Seeds into Your Diet

The versatility of chia seeds makes them easy to incorporate into a variety of meals. Here are some popular ways to enjoy these nutritional powerhouses:

Chia Pudding: Soak chia seeds in milk or a non-dairy alternative overnight. In the morning, add fruits, nuts, or sweeteners for a delicious and nutritious breakfast.

Smoothies: Add a tablespoon of chia seeds to your favorite smoothie for an extra boost of fiber, protein, and omega-3s.

Baking: Incorporate chia seeds into baked goods like muffins, bread, or pancakes for enhanced nutrition without sacrificing flavor.

Salads: Sprinkle chia seeds over salads for added crunch and nutrition.

Energy Bars: Mix chia seeds into homemade energy bars or granola for a healthy snack that curbs hunger.

As we have explored in this chapter, chia seeds truly earn their reputation as a "nutritional powerhouse." With their impressive array of nutrients, fiber, and antioxidants, they offer numerous health benefits that can enhance overall well-being. Whether you're looking to boost your heart health, support digestion, or simply add a nutritious twist to your meals, chia seeds serve as a convenient and versatile option.

Comparison with Other Seeds and Fibers

Fibers, on the other hand, provide a range of materials essential for clothing, textiles, and household goods. Understanding the nuances of various seeds and fibers allows for a greater appreciation of their benefits and limitations. This chapter aims to illuminate the similarities and differences among various seeds and fibers, providing a comprehensive overview of their characteristics, applications, and environmental implications.

1. Seeds: Nutritional Powerhouses ### 1.1. Common Seeds

Seeds, the reproductive units of flowering plants, come in many varieties. Some commonly used seeds include:

Sunflower Seeds: Rich in healthy fats and proteins, sunflower seeds are popular as snack foods, and seeds for retail, and are often incorporated into various culinary dishes.

Pumpkin Seeds: Also known as pepitas, these seeds are packed with magnesium, iron, and antioxidants, making them a popular choice for health-conscious consumers.

Flaxseeds: Known for their high omega-3 fatty acid content and dietary fiber, flaxseeds have gained attention as a superfood and are frequently used in smoothies, cereals, and nutritional supplements.

Chia Seeds: Similar to flaxseeds, chia seeds are heralded for their omega-3 content and ability to absorb water, forming a gel-like texture that is often used in puddings and health drinks.

1.2. Nutritional Comparison

When comparing these seeds, it is essential to consider their nutritional profiles. For instance, while sunflower seeds are rich in vitamin E and selenium, flaxseeds excel in omega-3 fatty acids and lignans, which have antioxidant properties. Chia seeds, on the other hand, stand out for their ability to retain moisture and provide a good source of fiber, making them beneficial for digestive health.

1.3. Economic and Cultivation Aspects

Economically, seeds such as sunflower and flax have established markets with significant demand in health food industries. The cultivation of these seeds varies widely, with sunflowers thriving in temperate climates and flax requiring specific soil conditions for optimal growth. Understanding these factors is crucial for farmers and investors considering the agricultural landscape.

2. Fibers: The Fabric of Society ### 2.1. Types of Fibers

Fibers, the elongated structures of varying lengths and strengths, are integral to countless products. Some primary sources of fiber include:

Cotton: The most widely used natural fiber, cotton is known for its softness, breathability, and versatility. It is predominantly used in apparel and textile manufacturing.

Hemp: Once stigmatized, hemp has resurfaced as a sustainable alternative to cotton and synthetic fibers. It is known for its strength, durability, and lower environmental impact.

Flax (Linen): Beyond being a nutritious seed source, flax fibers are extracted to produce linen, a textile appreciated for its natural luster and breathability.

Sisal: Derived from the agave plant, sisal fibers are strong and resistant, making them ideal for ropes, twine, and various biodegradable products.

2.2. Functional and Environmental Impact

When comparing these fibers, cotton is often critiqued for its heavy reliance on water and pesticides, raising sustainability concerns. Hemp and flax, conversely, typically require fewer resources and can improve soil health, making them environmentally friendly alternatives. However, hemp fibers can be coarse and may require blending with other materials for specific textile applications.

2.3. Economic Considerations

The fiber market is heavily influenced by consumer demand for sustainable products. As awareness of environmental impacts rises, the fiber industry is seeing a push towards alternatives like hemp and organic cotton. These shifts not only reflect changing consumer preferences but also indicate a broader movement towards sustainability in textiles.

3. Comparative Analysis: Seeds vs. Fibers ### 3.1. Nutritional vs. Structural Attributes

While seeds are primarily valued for their nutritional benefits, fibers are paramount for their structural attributes in creating modern textiles. The applications of each are distinctly different. Seeds serve as health supplements, while fibers form the backbone of the fashion and textiles industry.

3.2. Environmental Footprints

The production of both seeds and fibers carries an environmental footprint. Seed agriculture must balance the need for water, land, and pest control, while fiber production can challenge land use and sustainability practices. Here, the choice between cotton and hemp becomes crucial, as the latter presents a more environmentally sustainable profile.

3.3. Market Dynamics

Market dynamics for seeds and fibers also differ. Seeds have seen a rise in demand driven by health trends, whereas fibers are increasingly subjected to sustainability scrutiny and consumer awareness. Companies that embrace more sustainable practices are often rewarded with greater market share and consumer loyalty.

As agricultural practices continue to adapt, understanding the interplay between nutrition, economic viability, and environmental responsibility will be essential for the future of these indispensable products. The ongoing research and development in both sectors hold the promise of discovering more efficient and sustainable practices, ultimately leading us towards more responsible production and consumption patterns in a rapidly changing world.

How Chia Seeds Benefit Digestion

As people increasingly seek natural solutions to support their digestive health, superfoods like chia seeds have emerged as a popular choice. This chapter delves into the multifaceted ways in which chia seeds benefit digestion, making them a powerful ally in achieving optimal gut health.

The Nutritional Profile of Chia Seeds

Chia seeds (Salvia hispanica) are tiny black or white seeds harvested from the Salvia plant, native to Central America. These small powerhouses are packed with nutrients essential for digestive health:

High in Fiber: Chia seeds boast an impressive fiber content, with approximately 10 grams of fiber per ounce. This makes them an excellent food source for promoting healthy digestion.

Omega-3 Fatty Acids: Rich in alpha-linolenic acid (ALA), chia seeds provide anti-inflammatory benefits that can support gut health.

Protein: Containing around 4 grams of protein per ounce, chia seeds offer a plant-based protein source that aids in muscle health and can promote satiety.

Vitamins and Minerals: Chia seeds are loaded with various vitamins and minerals, including calcium, magnesium, and phosphorus, which are crucial for maintaining healthy bodily functions, including digestion.

Fiber: The Digestive Superstar

Chia seeds are primarily celebrated for their high fiber content, which significantly contributes to digestive health in several ways:

1. **Promotes Regularity**

Dietary fiber is a key component of a healthy digestive system. Chia seeds contain both soluble and insoluble fiber. Soluble fiber absorbs water and forms a gel-like substance, which helps to soften stool and make it easier to pass. Insoluble fiber adds bulk to stool, promoting regular bowel movements and preventing constipation. By incorporating chia seeds into your diet, you can help maintain a steady flow through your digestive tract, reducing the risk of digestive disruptions.

2. **Supports Gut Microbiota**

A healthy gut is home to trillions of microorganisms, collectively known as the gut microbiota, which plays a crucial role in digestion and overall health. Fibers, particularly prebiotics, serve as food for beneficial gut bacteria. Chia seeds are considered a prebiotic food source, nourishing these friendly bacteria and allowing them to flourish. A balanced gut microbiota can help improve digestion, fortify the immune system, and even influence mood.

3. **Helps Maintain a Healthy Weight**

The high fiber content in chia seeds also contributes to feelings of fullness and satiety. When mixed with liquid, chia seeds expand, creating a gel-like consistency that takes up space in the stomach. This helps curb appetite and can prevent overeating, which is a common culprit in digestive issues. Moreover, maintaining a healthy weight is essential, as excess weight can place additional stress on the digestive system.

Hydration and Digestive Health

Chia seeds have the unique ability to absorb water—up to 12 times their weight. This property plays a vital role in digestion:

1. **Aids Hydration**

Maintaining proper hydration is essential for effective digestion. When chia seeds are consumed with adequate water, they can help keep the digestive tract lubricated, promoting smoother bowel movements and preventing constipation. Staying well-hydrated can also flush out toxins and waste products, further supporting digestive health.

2. **Prevents Gastrointestinal Issues**

By absorbing water and creating a gel-like consistency, chia seeds can help create a more stable environment in the gut. This gel can help reduce symptoms of gastrointestinal discomfort, such as bloating and indigestion, by slowing the absorption of food, allowing for better digestion and nutrient absorption.

Anti-inflammatory Properties

Chronic inflammation can lead to a host of digestive issues, including disorders like Irritable Bowel Syndrome

(IBS) and inflammatory bowel disease (IBD). The omega-3 fatty acids present in chia seeds possess anti-inflammatory properties that can mitigate digestive inflammation, promoting a healthier gut environment. Consuming chia seeds regularly may help alleviate symptoms associated with these conditions, providing relief for those suffering from digestive discomfort.

Practical Ways to Incorporate Chia Seeds

Integrating chia seeds into your daily diet is simple and versatile. Here are some easy ideas to reap the digestive benefits they offer:

Chia Pudding: Combine chia seeds with almond milk or coconut milk, add a dash of sweetener and let it sit overnight in the refrigerator. Enjoy it in the morning as a nutrient-packed breakfast or snack.

Smoothies: Blend chia seeds into your favorite smoothie for an added fiber and nutrient boost.

Baking: Add chia seeds to muffins, bread, or pancake batter for extra texture and nutrition.

Soups and Stews: Sprinkle chia seeds into soups or stews as a thickening agent and nutritional enhancer.

Salads: Mix chia seeds into salad dressings or sprinkle them on top of salads for a satisfying crunch.

By incorporating them into your daily diet, you can pave the way—literally and figuratively—for smoother digestion and overall well-being. As we continue to explore the dynamic relationship between nutrition and gut health, chia seeds remain a simple yet impactful addition to our diets, redefining the conversation around digestive wellness in the modern world.

Chapter 3: Incorporating Chia Seeds into Your Diet

These tiny black or white seeds pack a powerful punch of nutritional benefits that can enhance any diet. With high levels of omega-3 fatty acids, fiber, antioxidants, and essential minerals, chia seeds offer a myriad of health advantages that warrant inclusion in your daily meals. This chapter will explore various ways to easily incorporate chia seeds into your diet, allowing you to enjoy their health benefits daily.

Understanding the Nutritional Benefits

Before diving into practical applications, it is essential to understand what makes chia seeds so beneficial. With a remarkable nutrient profile, chia seeds are considered a superfood. Each ounce (about two tablespoons) contains approximately:

139 calories

9 grams of fat (mostly polyunsaturated)

11 grams of carbohydrates

10 grams of fiber

4 grams of protein

Minerals like calcium, manganese, magnesium, phosphorus, and zinc

The high fiber content aids digestion, supports gut health, and helps maintain a sense of fullness, making chia seeds an excellent choice for weight management. Additionally, their omega-3 fatty acids contribute to heart health, while their antioxidants combat oxidative stress, promoting overall wellness.

Easy Ways to Add Chia Seeds to Your Meals ### 1. Chia Pudding

One of the most popular and delicious ways to incorporate chia seeds into your diet is by making chia pudding. It's simple to prepare and can be customized to suit your taste.

Basic Chia Pudding Recipe:

Ingredients:

1/4 cup chia seeds

1 cup almond milk (or any milk of your choice)

1 tablespoon sweetener (honey, maple syrup, or stevia)

1/2 teaspoon vanilla extract (optional)

Instructions:

In a bowl or jar, mix chia seeds, almond milk, sweetener, and vanilla extract until combined.

Cover and refrigerate for at least 3 hours or overnight.

Stir again before serving, and enjoy with fresh fruits, nuts, or granola as toppings. ### 2. Smoothies

Chia seeds are an excellent addition to smoothies, adding texture and nutritional density. Simply toss a tablespoon or two into your blender along with your favorite fruits, leafy greens, and liquid base.

Example Smoothie Recipe:

1 banana

1/2 cup spinach

1 tablespoon chia seeds

1 cup coconut water or almond milk

Blend until smooth, and enjoy a refreshing, nutrient-packed beverage! ### 3. Baking

Chia seeds can also be incorporated into baked goods. Add them to muffins, bread, or pancakes for an extra boost of nutrition.

Tip: Replace a portion of the flour in your recipes with ground chia seeds, or add whole seeds to the batter for a delightful crunch.

4. Salads

Sprinkle chia seeds over salads for added texture and nutrition. They can also be mixed into salad dressings or marinades to enhance flavor and nutritional content.

Chia Seed Dressing:

1/4 cup olive oil

2 tablespoons apple cider vinegar

1 tablespoon chia seeds

Salt and pepper to taste

Combine in a jar, shake well, and drizzle over your favorite salad. ### 5. Energy Bites

Creating energy bites or bars filled with chia seeds is another fantastic way to incorporate them into your diet. You can mix them with oats, nut butter, honey, and any other ingredients you have on hand.

Basic Energy Bite Recipe:

Ingredients:

1 cup rolled oats

1/2 cup nut butter

1/4 cup honey or maple syrup

1/4 cup chia seeds

Optional add-ins: chocolate chips, dried fruits, or nuts

Instructions:

Combine all ingredients in a bowl and mix well.

Form the mixture into small balls and refrigerate for at least 30 minutes.

Store in an airtight container in the fridge for quick, nutritious snacks on the go. ### 6. Soups and Stews

Chia seeds can be added to soups or stews as a thickening agent. They not only add nutritional value but also give your dishes a wholesome texture.

7. Hydration

Chia seeds are known for their ability to absorb water, swelling up to ten times their size. To create a refreshing drink, soak chia seeds in water or fruit juice for 20-30 minutes, then stir and enjoy. This will not only keep you hydrated but also provide a satisfying texture.

Incorporating chia seeds into your diet can be done with ease and creativity. With their subtle flavor, these versatile seeds can be added to an array of dishes, enhancing both nutrition and taste. Whether you choose to make a refreshing pudding, blend them into a smoothie, or simply sprinkle them over your meals, chia seeds can provide a health boost with every bite.

Easy Ways to Add Chia Seeds to Meals

Whether you're a seasoned chia enthusiast or someone curious about incorporating these superfoods into your meals, this chapter will explore easy and delicious methods to flavorfully and healthfully add chia seeds to your everyday recipes.

Understanding Chia Seeds

Before diving into the various ways to use chia seeds, it's important to understand their unique properties. When soaked in liquid, chia seeds can absorb up to twelve times their weight, forming a gel-like consistency. This quality makes them not only a great source of hydration but also a satisfying addition to meals that enhances texture.

1. Smoothies

One of the simplest ways to incorporate chia seeds into your diet is by adding them to smoothies. Their neutral flavor won't overpower your favorite combinations, and they can boost the nutritional value significantly.

How to Use:

Simply add one to two tablespoons of chia seeds to your blender when making a smoothie.

For a variety in texture, let the seeds soak in a little water for 15 minutes before blending. This will ensure a thicker consistency.

Suggested Combination:

Spinach, banana, almond milk, and a tablespoon of chia seeds make for a nutritious, energy-boosting start to your day.

2. Overnight Oats

Overnight oats are an excellent breakfast choice that can easily be enhanced with chia seeds. They provide extra fiber and help to keep you full until lunch.

How to Use:

In a jar, mix together rolled oats, milk (or a milk alternative), sweetener, and chia seeds.

Let the mixture sit overnight in the fridge, letting the chia seeds absorb the liquid and expand.

Suggested Recipe:

Combine 1/2 cup rolled oats, 1 tablespoon chia seeds, 1 cup almond milk, and 1 tablespoon of maple syrup. Add toppings like fresh fruit, nuts, or granola in the morning.

3. Baking

Chia seeds can also be incorporated into baked goods, adding nutrition and a subtle crunch. ### How to Use:

Substitute a portion of the flour in your recipes with ground chia seeds or add whole seeds to enhance texture in muffins, bread, or pancakes.

Suggested Recipe:

For chia seed muffins, combine 1 cup of flour, 1/4 cup ground chia seeds, 1/2 cup oats, 1/2 cup sugar, and 1/4 cup chia seeds. Mix in wet ingredients like mashed banana and almond milk, then bake. ## 4. Salads

Sprinkling chia seeds over salads is a fantastic way to boost your meal's nutritional content without altering the flavor significantly.

How to Use:

Simply sprinkle a tablespoon of chia seeds over salads just before serving for an extra crunch and nutrition boost.

Suggested Combination:

A spinach salad with cherry tomatoes, cucumber, feta cheese, walnuts, and a sprinkle of chia seeds offers great texture and an omega-3 punch.

5. Pudding

Chia seed pudding is a versatile dessert that can be flavored in numerous ways, making it a favorite among health enthusiasts.

How to Use:

Combine chia seeds with your choice of milk and a sweetener, let it sit for several hours or overnight, and enjoy it plain or topped with fruits and nuts.

Basic Chia Seed Pudding Recipe:

Mix together 1/4 cup chia seeds, 1 cup almond milk, and 1 tablespoon maple syrup. Stir well and refrigerate until it thickens.

Flavor Variations:

Add vanilla extract, cocoa powder, or matcha for different flavors. ## 6. Soups and Sauces

Chia seeds can also be used as a natural thickening agent

in soups and sauces.

How to Use:

Stir in a tablespoon of chia seeds to your soup or sauce while cooking; they'll help thicken the mixture without altering the flavor.

Suggested Dish:

A creamy tomato soup can benefit from chia seeds, giving it additional nutrients while maintaining its smooth texture.

7. Energy Bars and Snacks

DIY energy bars made from nuts, dried fruits, and chia seeds make for a healthy grab-and-go snack. ### How to Use:

Blend together your choice of nuts, dates, and fibers with chia seeds, then press the mixture into a pan and refrigerate.

Simple Recipe:

Blend 1 cup of mixed nuts, 1 cup of dates, and 1/4 cup of chia seeds until combined. Press into a lined pan, refrigerate, and cut into bars.

As you experiment and explore, you'll soon discover that incorporating chia seeds can turn even the simplest dishes into healthful delights. So grab a bag of chia seeds and start adding them to your meals; your body will thank you!

Creative Uses for Chia Seeds

While many know them primarily as a nutritious addition to smoothies or oatmeal, their versatility allows for a plethora of innovative and unexpected applications. In this chapter, we will explore some of the most creative uses for chia seeds that go beyond the conventional.

1. Chia Seed Pudding

Perhaps the most well-known way to enjoy chia seeds is through chia seed pudding, a delightful dish that serves as a nutritious breakfast or a satisfying dessert. By combining chia seeds with your choice of milk or plant-based milk (coconut, almond, oat), along with a sweetener like honey or maple syrup, and letting the mixture sit in the refrigerator for a few hours or overnight, you'll create a creamy, custard-like delight. Jazz it up by incorporating vanilla extract, cocoa powder, or fresh fruit. The possibilities are endless, allowing for seasonal flavors that can cater to every taste preference.

2. A Substitute for Eggs

For those following a vegan or egg-free lifestyle, chia seeds can serve as a fantastic egg substitute in baking. By mixing one tablespoon of chia seeds with three tablespoons of water and letting it sit until it forms a gel- like consistency, you'll have a binder that works wonders in recipes like muffins, pancakes, and cookies.

This innovative use not only enhances the texture of baked goods but also adds nutritional value. ## 3. Hydrating Drinks

Chia seeds can transform a regular beverage into an energizing health booster. When soaked in water, they absorb liquid, developing a unique gel-like texture. This makes them a perfect addition to wellness drinks. Try adding soaked chia seeds to lemon water for an invigorating drink full of electrolytes, or incorporate them into smoothies for extra thickness and nutrition. In some cultures, chia seeds are even used in traditional drinks like "chia fresca," where they are mixed with water, lime juice, and a sweetener for a refreshing treat.

4. Breakfast Toppers

Chia seeds are great as a topping on various breakfast favorites. Sprinkle them over your morning yogurt, oatmeal, or cereal for an added health boost. Their crunchy texture complements fruits, nuts, and granola, creating a balanced and fulfilling meal that keeps you satisfied longer. You can also blend them into smoothies for a creamy finish or use them to garnish smoothie bowls, creating a visually appealing and nutritious breakfast.

5. Chia Jam

Making your own chia jam could be one of the most delectable and creative uses for chia seeds. By combining fresh or frozen fruit with chia seeds and a natural sweetener, you can whip up a quick and easy jam that contains no preservatives. The chia seeds not only provide texture to the jam but also act as a thickening agent. Simmer your fruit until soft, stir in the chia seeds, and let the mixture cool. You'll be left with a delicious, homemade jam perfect for spreading on toast or adding to desserts.

6. Healthy Salads

Incorporating chia seeds into salads is an excellent way to add crunch and health benefits. They can be sprinkled on top of leafy greens or mixed into dressings to create a nutrient-dense meal. A delightful option is to create a chia vinaigrette, where you blend olive oil, vinegar, garlic, and soaked chia seeds. This dressing not only enhances flavor but also helps to thicken the dressing, allowing it to cling beautifully to your salad ingredients.

7. Energy Bites and Bars

Busy lifestyles call for quick sources of energy, and chia seeds can easily be incorporated into homemade energy bites or bars. Combining oats, nut butter, honey, or agave syrup along with chia seeds, you can form bite-sized pieces that are both nutritious and satisfying. These energy bites provide an excellent source of sustained energy, making them perfect for pre-workout snacks or mid-afternoon fuel.

8. Chia Seed Breads

For the adventurous baker, incorporating chia seeds into homemade bread recipes can yield delicious results. Chia seeds can be mixed into bread, giving it a unique texture and acting as a natural egg substitute. You can also make a gluten-free version using nut flours, chia seeds, and a bit of water. This is a great way to increase your fiber intake while enjoying a fresh loaf of bread.

9. Homemade Granola

If you enjoy granola, consider adding chia seeds for extra crunch and nutrition. Mixing them into your homemade granola recipe can elevate its health benefits, making it a powerhouse breakfast option. Combine rolled oats, nuts, seeds, honey (or maple syrup), and a generous sprinkle of chia seeds, then bake until golden brown. You'll have a delightful snack or breakfast option that packs a nutrient punch.

Chapter 4: Managing IBS Symptoms with Chia Seeds

A particularly promising food in this context is chia seeds. This chapter delves into the potential benefits of incorporating chia seeds into the diets of those suffering from IBS, exploring their nutritional properties, practical applications, and tips for using them effectively to manage symptoms.

Understanding IBS and Dietary Interventions

IBS is characterized by its chronic nature, with common triggers including stress, food intolerances, and changes in gut microbiota. While there is no one-size-fits-all solution for managing IBS, dietary modifications often play a significant role in symptom control. Many individuals find relief through low-FODMAP diets, high-fiber foods, and the inclusion of specific seeds and grains that promote digestive health. Chia seeds, in particular, are gaining attention for their unique combination of fiber, omega-3 fatty acids, and antioxidants.

The Nutritional Profile of Chia Seeds

Chia seeds are small white or black seeds derived from the *Salvia hispanica* plant, native to Central America. They have gained popularity in recent years due to their impressive nutritional profile, which includes:

High Fiber Content: Chia seeds are rich in both soluble

and insoluble fiber. This is important for individuals with IBS, as fiber helps regulate bowel movements and can alleviate both diarrhea and constipation.

Omega-3 Fatty Acids: These essential fats are known for their anti-inflammatory properties, potentially beneficial for individuals whose IBS symptoms are exacerbated by inflammation.

Antioxidants: Chia seeds are packed with antioxidants, which can help combat oxidative stress and inflammation in the body.

Protein: They also contain a good amount of plant-based protein, which can help maintain muscle mass and overall health.

How Chia Seeds Help Manage IBS Symptoms

1. Promoting Digestive Health

The soluble fiber in chia seeds forms a gel-like substance when combined with liquid. This gel can help soften stool, making it easier to pass and reducing the likelihood of constipation. For individuals with diarrhea-predominant IBS, the gel-like consistency can also help increase stool bulk, as soluble fiber absorbs excess water in the intestines.

2. Reducing Inflammation

The omega-3 fatty acids found in chia seeds may help reduce intestinal inflammation, potentially calming some of the underlying issues that trigger IBS symptoms. By including chia seeds in their diet, individuals with IBS may find a reduction in bloating and discomfort after meals.

3. Enhancing Gut Health

Chia seeds have prebiotic properties, meaning they can support the growth of healthy gut bacteria. A balanced gut microbiome is vital for digestion and can be particularly beneficial for individuals suffering from IBS, as an imbalanced microbiota may exacerbate symptoms.

4. Stabilizing Blood Sugar Levels

Incorporating chia seeds into meals can help stabilize blood sugar levels. Fluctuating blood sugar can affect digestive health, so the slow release of energy provided by chia seeds may assist in maintaining a more even energy and digestion flow.

Practical Ways to Incorporate Chia Seeds into Your Diet

Incorporating chia seeds into your diet can be simple and versatile. Here are some practical ways to do so: ### Chia Pudding

Chia pudding is a popular and delicious way to enjoy chia seeds. Combine chia seeds with your choice of milk (dairy or plant-based) and a sweetener of your choice. Let the mixture sit for several hours or overnight to allow it to thicken. Top with fruits, nuts, or flavorings like vanilla or cocoa for added taste.

Smoothies

Add a tablespoon of chia seeds to your morning smoothie for a nutritional boost. Blend them alongside your favorite fruits, leafy greens, and a source of protein for a filling meal that supports digestive health.

Sprinkling on Salads and Bowls

Chia seeds can be sprinkled onto salads, grain bowls, or yogurt. Their mild flavor makes them a perfect addition without altering the taste of your dish.

Baked Goods

Incorporate chia seeds into muffins, pancakes, or bread. They can enhance texture and nutrition while providing health benefits.

Tips for Using Chia Seeds in IBS Management

Start Slowly: If you are new to chia seeds, begin with a small amount, as increasing fiber intake too quickly can initially exacerbate IBS symptoms for some people.

Stay Hydrated: Since chia seeds absorb liquid, it is vital to drink plenty of water throughout the day to stay hydrated and support digestive health.

Monitor Your Body's Response: Keep a food diary to track any changes in symptoms as you introduce chia seeds into your diet. This can help identify how your body reacts to different quantities and preparations.

By incorporating this nutrient-rich seed into your diet, you can take proactive steps toward better digestive health. However, as with any dietary change, it is essential to consult with a healthcare professional or a registered dietitian, especially if IBS symptoms are severe or persistent. Embrace the power of chia seeds and explore the myriad ways they can enrich your meals and support your journey to better health.

Relieving Constipation Naturally

While over-the-counter medications can offer quick relief, many individuals prefer to explore natural remedies to alleviate their discomfort and promote regularity. This chapter will delve into various natural methods for relieving constipation, focusing on dietary changes, lifestyle modifications, herbal remedies, and holistic approaches.

Understanding Constipation

Before addressing how to relieve constipation naturally, it's important to understand what constipation is. Defined as infrequent bowel movements or difficulty in passing stools, constipation can be caused by a variety of factors, including poor diet, dehydration, lack of physical activity, stress, and certain medical conditions. Symptoms may include abdominal pain, bloating, and a sense of incomplete evacuation.

Dietary Changes

Increase Fiber Intake

One of the most effective ways to relieve constipation naturally is by increasing fiber intake. Dietary fiber adds bulk to the stool and helps it pass more easily through the intestines. There are two types of fiber—soluble and insoluble—both of which play a role in digestive health.

Soluble Fiber: Found in oats, beans, lentils, and fruits such as apples and citrus, soluble fiber absorbs water and forms a gel-like substance, which can help soften stools.

Insoluble Fiber: Found in whole grains, nuts, vegetables, and wheat bran, insoluble fiber adds bulk to the stool and promotes movement through the digestive tract.

Aiming for a daily intake of 25 to 30 grams of fiber is ideal. To increase fiber gradually, introduce high-fiber foods into your diet, such as whole grains, fruits, and vegetables, and combine them with adequate hydration.

Stay Hydrated

Adequate hydration is paramount in preventing and relieving constipation. Water plays a crucial role in softening stool and facilitating movement through the intestines. Aim for at least 8 cups (64 ounces) of water daily, but remember that individual needs may vary based on activity level and climate.

Incorporate Probiotics

Probiotics are beneficial bacteria that promote gut health and can enhance digestive function. Foods rich in probiotics include yogurt, kefir, sauerkraut, kimchi, and other fermented foods. These foods may help regulate bowel movements and prevent constipation. Consider adding a probiotic supplement to your routine, particularly if you're experiencing persistent digestive issues.

Lifestyle Modifications ### Regular Exercise

Physical activity is essential for maintaining a healthy digestive system. Regular exercise stimulates intestinal contractions, which can help move stools through the colon. Aim for at least 150 minutes of moderate aerobic activity each week, along with strength training exercises on two or more days. Simple activities like walking, jogging, or yoga can significantly contribute to improved bowel function.

Establish a Routine

Establishing a regular bathroom routine can help train your body. Try to visit the bathroom at the same time each day, allowing yourself enough time to relax and avoid feeling rushed. Listening to your body's cues is key; when you feel the urge to go, don't ignore it.

Manage Stress

Stress and anxiety can negatively affect digestive health, leading to constipation. Practicing stress management techniques—such as mindfulness, meditation, deep breathing exercises, and yoga—can help ease tension and promote healthy bowel function.

Herbal Remedies ### Senna

Senna is a natural laxative made from the leaves and fruit of the senna plant. It is commonly used in herbal remedies to support bowel movements. However, it should be used judiciously and not as a long-term solution, as regular use may lead to dependence on laxatives.

Psyllium Husk

Psyllium husk is a soluble fiber that can help regulate bowel movements and alleviate constipation. It works by absorbing water and forming a gel-like substance, which can soften stools and promote their passage. Be sure to consume enough fluids when taking psyllium to avoid potential blockages.

Flaxseeds

Flaxseeds are rich in both soluble and insoluble fiber, making them an excellent choice for promoting digestive health. Ground flaxseeds can be added to smoothies, yogurt, or baked goods for a nutritious boost, helping to relieve constipation.

Holistic Approaches ### Acupressure

Acupressure, an ancient Chinese medicine technique, may provide relief for constipation symptoms. Certain pressure points, such as the large intestine 4 (LI4) point located between the thumb and index finger, can stimulate bowel activity. Applying gentle pressure to these points for several minutes may encourage regular bowel movements.

Abdominal Massage

Gentle abdominal massage can help stimulate the digestive system and relieve bloating and discomfort. Use circular motions with your fingers, starting at the lower right side of your abdomen and moving in a clockwise direction. This technique can promote peristalsis and help move stool through the intestines.

Relieving constipation naturally focuses on fostering a healthy lifestyle and making dietary adjustments rather than relying solely on pharmacological solutions. By incorporating high-fiber foods, staying hydrated, getting regular exercise, managing stress, and exploring herbal remedies, individuals can achieve a more regular and comfortable digestive routine.

Reducing Inflammation and Bloating with chia seeds

Fortunately, nature provides us with a wealth of resources to help combat these challenges, and one such superfood that has gained significant attention in recent years is chia seeds. Known for their nutritional prowess, these tiny seeds pack a powerful punch when it comes to reducing inflammation and alleviating bloating. This chapter explores the science behind chia seeds, their health benefits, and practical ways to incorporate them into your diet for digestive wellness.

Understanding Inflammation and Bloating

Before delving into the benefits of chia seeds, it's essential to comprehend the issues at hand. Inflammation is a natural response of the body to protect itself from injury or infection. However, when it becomes chronic due to factors like poor diet, stress, and environmental toxins, it can lead to a host of health problems including heart disease, diabetes, and autoimmune disorders. Similarly, bloating—often a sign of digestive distress—can result from various factors including excess gas, food intolerances, and imbalances in gut bacteria.

Bringing attention to these issues raises the question: how can we harness the power of chia seeds to help manage and mitigate these conditions?

The Nutritional Breakdown of Chia Seeds

Chia seeds are tiny, oval-shaped seeds that come from the Salvia hispanica plant, originating in Central and South America. They are a rich source of nutrients that contribute to their anti-inflammatory properties and digestive support:

Omega-3 Fatty Acids: Chia seeds are one of the richest plant sources of omega-3 fatty acids, particularly alpha-linolenic acid (ALA). Omega-3s are known for their ability to decrease inflammation in the body, making them vital for individuals dealing with inflammatory conditions.

Fiber: Chia seeds are packed with soluble fiber, which can help promote regular bowel movements and mitigate bloating. This fiber forms a gel-like substance when mixed with water, slowing down digestion and providing a feeling of fullness.

Antioxidants: Chia seeds contain a plethora of antioxidants, which can help combat oxidative stress in the body, reducing inflammation and promoting cellular health.

Minerals: These seeds are an excellent source of essential minerals such as magnesium, calcium, and phosphorus, which play crucial roles in maintaining bone health and proper metabolic function.

How Chia Seeds Combat Inflammation

Several studies have shown that incorporating chia seeds into your diet can help reduce markers of inflammation in the body. Omega-3 fatty acids, in particular, have been linked to lowered levels of inflammatory cytokines. Regular consumption of chia seeds can help balance the omega-3 to omega-6 fatty acid ratio in the diet, reducing systemic inflammation.

Furthermore, the high fiber content in chia seeds contributes to gut health by feeding beneficial gut bacteria and promoting regularity. A healthy gut microbiome is essential for managing inflammation since a balanced

microbial community can help regulate immune responses and inflammation in the body. ## Alleviating Bloating with Chia Seeds

Bloating can often be traced back to digestive issues, such as gut dysbiosis, food sensitivities, or simply consuming foods that are hard to digest. Chia seeds can provide relief in the following ways:

Soaking and Gel Formation: When chia seeds are soaked in liquid, they expand and form a gel-like consistency. This gel can slow down the digestion of carbohydrates and fats, allowing for better absorption of nutrients and reducing the occurrence of bloating.

Improved Digestion: The soluble fiber in chia seeds aids in the movement of food through the digestive tract, helping to reduce constipation and the discomfort associated with bloating.

Hydration: Chia seeds absorb up to 12 times their weight in water, making them an excellent choice for maintaining hydration. Proper hydration is crucial for optimal digestive function, helping to prevent constipation and reduce bloating.

Practical Tips for Incorporating Chia Seeds into Your Diet

Incorporating chia seeds into your daily routine is simple and versatile. Here are some easy ways to enjoy their benefits:

Chia Pudding: One of the most popular ways to enjoy chia seeds is by making chia pudding. Combine chia seeds with your choice of milk (dairy or plant-based) and sweetener, allow it to sit for a few hours or overnight, and enjoy it as a nutritious breakfast or snack.

Smoothies: Add a tablespoon of chia seeds to your smoothies for a boost of nutrition and a thicker texture. They pair well with fruits, vegetables, and yogurt.

Baking: Incorporate chia seeds into your baked goods by adding them to muffins, bread, or cookies. They not only enhance the nutrient profile but also add a pleasant crunch.

Salads and Soups: Sprinkle chia seeds on salads or stir them into soups for added texture and nutrition. They also work well as a topping for yogurt or oatmeal.

Energy Bars and Snacks: Chia seeds can be a great addition to homemade energy bars or snack mixes, providing a healthy dose of fiber and protein.

Chia seeds are more than just a trendy health food; they are a nutrient-dense superfood that can play a significant role in reducing inflammation and alleviating bloating. Rich in omega-3 fatty acids, fiber, and antioxidants, chia seeds support gut health and provide relief from digestive discomfort.

Chapter 5: Expert Advice on Using Chia Seeds for IBS

While there is no one-size-fits-all solution for treating IBS, dietary options play a crucial role in alleviating symptoms. In this chapter, we will explore the potential benefits of incorporating chia seeds into your diet, along with expert tips on how to use them effectively for those suffering from IBS.

Understanding Chia Seeds

Chia seeds, derived from the *Salvia hispanica* plant, are a powerhouse of nutrients. They are rich in omega-3 fatty acids, dietary fiber, protein, and various essential minerals. When soaked in water, chia seeds form a gel-like substance due to their high soluble fiber content, which can be beneficial for digestive health.

For individuals with IBS, it is essential to maintain a balance between soluble and insoluble fiber. Soluble fiber can help regulate bowel movements by absorbing water and forming a gel-like consistency, while insoluble fiber adds bulk to stool and helps it pass through the intestines more quickly. The soluble fiber in chia seeds can be especially advantageous for those with diarrhea-predominant IBS (IBS-D) or a mixed subtype of the condition.

Benefits of Chia Seeds for IBS

Promotes Regularity: The soluble fiber in chia seeds can help regulate bowel movements by absorbing excess water and forming soft stool consistency, making them particularly beneficial for individuals with IBS-D.

Hydration Support: Chia seeds can absorb up to 12 times their weight in water, helping to keep the digestive tract hydrated and potentially reducing constipation in individuals with constipation-predominant IBS (IBS-C).

Gut Health: The prebiotic properties of chia seeds can promote the growth of beneficial gut bacteria, contributing to overall gut health and potentially reducing IBS symptoms.

Anti-Inflammatory Properties: The omega-3 fatty acids in chia seeds have anti-inflammatory properties, which may be beneficial for individuals with IBS, as inflammation often plays a role in the condition.

Expert Tips for Incorporating Chia Seeds into Your Diet

1. Start Slow: If you are new to using chia seeds, it's important to start with small amounts to assess how your body reacts. Begin with one teaspoon (5 grams) per day and gradually increase to 1 or 2 tablespoons (15 to 30 grams) based on your tolerance.

2. Hydration is Key: Always soak chia seeds in liquid before consuming them. For optimal results, use a 1:6 ratio (one part chia seeds to six parts liquid). This can be water, coconut water, almond milk, or even fruit juice. Let the mixture sit for at least 15 minutes (or longer) until it reaches a gel-like consistency.

3. Add Them to Smoothies and Yogurt: Chia seeds can be a great addition to smoothies or yogurt. They enhance the texture and nutritional value without significantly altering the flavor. Combine them with gut-friendly ingredients like bananas, spinach, or low-sugar yogurt to create a balanced meal.

4. Use as a Thickener: Chia seeds can serve as a natural thickening agent in soups, sauces, and dressings. Their ability to absorb water and expand can enhance the texture and nutritional profile of these foods.

5. Experiment with Chia Pudding: Create a chia pudding by mixing soaked chia seeds with coconut milk or almond milk and adding natural sweeteners and spices like cinnamon or vanilla. Let it sit in the fridge overnight for a delicious and filling breakfast option.

6. Monitor Your Symptoms: Keep a food diary to track your symptoms in relation to chia seed intake. This will help you identify what works best for you and allow for adjustments based on how your body responds.

Caution and Considerations

While chia seeds offer numerous benefits, they may not be suitable for everyone. Some individuals with IBS may still experience discomfort if they consume excessive amounts of fiber too quickly. Additionally, those with a history of choking or swallowing difficulties should be cautious, as chia seeds can expand rapidly in the throat.

It's also vital to consult with a healthcare professional or dietitian before making significant dietary changes, particularly if you have specific concerns related to IBS. They can provide personalized recommendations based on your unique symptoms and nutritional needs.

Incorporating chia seeds into your diet can be a simple yet effective strategy for managing symptoms of IBS. With their rich nutritional profile and versatility, chia seeds can enhance various meals and snacks while promoting gut health. However, the journey to managing IBS is individualized, and it's essential to listen to your body and make well-informed dietary choices. With expert guidance and mindful experimentation, you may find that chia seeds become a valuable ally in your quest for relief.

The importance of seeking a specialist to identify the problem of constipation

While occasional constipation may be a minor inconvenience, persistent cases can severely affect an individual's quality of life. Despite its prevalence, many individuals may not realize the importance of consulting a specialist for a proper diagnosis and effective treatment. This chapter will delve into the significance of seeking specialist care for constipation, the potential underlying issues that may contribute to the condition, and the benefits of a targeted approach to treatment.

Understanding Constipation

Before discussing the importance of specialists, it is essential to understand what constipation truly entails. The common medical definition indicates that constipation refers to infrequent bowel movements or difficulty in passing

Definition aside, constipation can manifest in various ways. Some individuals may experience alternating bouts of constipation and diarrhea, while others may grapple with chronic and long-standing issues. In seeking an understanding of constipation, it is crucial to recognize that it can be symptomatic of various underlying conditions—from dietary imbalances to more complex gastrointestinal disorders.

The Role of Specialists

When confronted with constipation, many individuals may initially seek advice from general practitioners, over-the-counter remedies, or lifestyle adjustments aimed at dietary changes and increased hydration. While these measures can be helpful for mild or sporadic issues, a specialist often possesses the expertise necessary to identify more intricate medical causes.

Identifying Underlying Conditions

Constipation can be symptomatic of a range of complications, including:

Irritable Bowel Syndrome (IBS): A functional gastrointestinal disorder that can lead to altered bowel habits, including constipation.

Metabolic Disorders: Thyroid dysfunction or diabetes can disrupt regular bowel function, leading to constipation.

Neurological Disorders: Conditions such as multiple sclerosis or Parkinson's disease can affect the nerves that help control bowel movements.

Structural Abnormalities: Issues such as pelvic floor dysfunction or colon obstruction require specialized knowledge for diagnosis and treatment.

Consulting a specialist, such as a gastroenterologist or a colorectal surgeon, is vital as they have access to advanced diagnostic tools and techniques—such as colonoscopy or motility studies—that can help pinpoint the root cause of constipation.

Comprehensive Evaluation

A specialist's approach to constipation is holistic and patient-centered, often beginning with a thorough evaluation of medical history, lifestyle, dietary habits, and symptoms. This comprehensive assessment may include:

Detailed Symptom History: Understanding when the constipation started, its frequency, and various accompanying symptoms.

Medications Review: Evaluating current medications to see if they contribute to constipation.

Diagnostic Tests: Recommending blood tests, imaging studies, or stool tests to get a clearer picture.

A detailed evaluation allows specialists to craft customized treatment strategies rather than relying on generic, one-size-fits-all solutions.

Benefits of Specialized Treatment

Seeking specialized care for constipation offers several benefits:

Targeted Treatment Plans: Specialists are equipped to devise targeted treatment plans that address the specific causes of constipation, rather than merely offering symptomatic relief.

Access to Advanced Therapies: Patients may benefit from cutting-edge therapies not typically offered in primary care settings. These can include biofeedback therapy, medications designed for chronic constipation, or minimally invasive surgical options.

Education and Support: Specialists can provide education on the condition, including dietary recommendations, lifestyle modifications, and an understanding of bowel health. This knowledge empowers patients to manage their condition effectively and prevent future episodes.

Long-Term Management: Chronic constipation often requires ongoing care and monitoring. Specialists can create long-term management plans that adapt as the patient's needs evolve.

Constipation, though common, can be the symptom of something much more complex lurking beneath the surface. In an era where individuals can often rely on quick fixes and over-the-counter medications, it is crucial to acknowledge the importance of consulting a specialist when faced with persistent or severe constipation.

Integrating Chia Seeds with Other Constipation Treatments

The discomfort associated with this condition can significantly impact one's quality of life. While various treatments are available, the incorporation of dietary components, such as chia seeds, has gained attention for their potential benefits in alleviating constipation. This chapter explores how chia seeds can be effectively integrated with other constipation treatments to optimize digestive health.

Understanding Chia Seeds

Chia seeds, derived from the Salvia hispanica plant, are small, nutrient-dense seeds that have been used for centuries. They are particularly high in soluble fiber, omega-3 fatty acids, protein, and various essential minerals such as calcium, magnesium, and phosphorus. When hydrated, chia seeds form a gel-like substance that can aid in increasing stool bulk and promoting regularity. They have become increasingly popular not only for their nutritional benefits but also for their ability to enhance digestive health.

The Role of Fiber in Constipation

Fiber is an essential component of a healthy diet and plays a pivotal role in digestive health. It can be classified into two main types: soluble and insoluble fiber.

Soluble fiber dissolves in water and forms a gel-like substance, which helps to slow digestion and absorb nutrients. It is beneficial for people experiencing constipation as it adds bulk to the stool and facilitates smoother passage.

Insoluble fiber, found in whole grains, nuts, and vegetables, aids in adding bulk to the stool and helps to promote movement through the digestive tract.

Chia seeds are unique in that they contain both types of fiber, making them a powerful ally in managing constipation. However, to achieve the best results, it's important to integrate chia seeds with other treatments effectively.

Integrating Chia Seeds with Dietary Modifications

Increase Water Intake

One of the most important adjustments when incorporating chia seeds into a diet is the increase in water intake. Chia seeds can absorb up to ten times their weight in water, which can lead to dehydration if not consumed with adequate fluids. For best results, aim to consume chia seeds soaked in water, smoothies, or other liquid-based dishes. This ensures that their fiber can work effectively without contributing to further constipation.

Combine with Other High-Fiber Foods

To maximize the benefits of chia seeds, consider integrating them with other high-fiber foods. Foods such as fruits (like apples, pears, and berries), vegetables (like leafy greens and carrots), legumes (like lentils and beans), and whole grains (like oats and quinoa) can enhance overall fiber intake. For example, adding chia seeds to a morning bowl of oatmeal dotted with berries elevates both the nutritional profile and fiber content of the meal.

Balanced Diet and Regular Meals

A balanced diet consisting of whole, minimally processed foods plays a crucial role in establishing regular bowel habits. Chia seeds can serve as a convenient topping or ingredient in various dishes, contributing to a daily regimen that includes regular, balanced meals. Strategies like meal prepping and planning can ensure that individuals have easy access to fiber-rich meals, including those featuring chia seeds.

Integrating Chia Seeds with Lifestyle Changes ### Physical Activity

In addition to dietary changes, physical activity is an

important component of managing constipation. Regular exercise stimulates digestive processes and enhance overall gut health. Chia seeds can serve as a convenient source of energy and nutrition before or after workouts. For instance, a chia seed pudding topped with fruits can be a nutritious pre- or post-workout snack, helping to stimulate digestion while providing sustained energy.

Mindful Eating

Practicing mindful eating—paying attention to hunger cues, savoring food, and chewing slowly—can help improve digestion and leads to healthier eating habits. Incorporating chia seeds into meals can encourage individuals to be more deliberate about their food choices. Consider adding chia seeds to salads or smoothies while taking time to enjoy the flavors and textures in each bite.

Integrating Chia Seeds with Medical Treatments ### Over-the-Counter (OTC) Laxatives

While chia seeds offer natural relief, individuals suffering from chronic constipation may rely on over-the- counter laxatives as part of their regimen. It is essential to consult a healthcare provider before combining chia seeds with laxatives, as certain laxatives may interact adversely with high-fiber foods. However, chia seeds can often complement the use of fiber-based laxatives by enhancing stool consistency and promoting regularity.

Probiotic Supplements

Probiotics—beneficial bacteria that support gut health— can be used in conjunction with chia seeds. Evidence suggests that probiotics may improve overall gut function and help alleviate constipation. Incorporating probiotic-rich foods such as yogurt, kefir, or fermented vegetables alongside chia seeds can yield synergistic effects, enhancing digestion and overall well-being.

As with any treatment, it is crucial to listen to one's body, stay hydrated, and consult with healthcare professionals to determine the best strategy for individual needs. Embracing a holistic approach that includes chia seeds may pave the way for improved digestive health and overall wellness.

Chapter 6: Creating a Balanced IBS Diet Plan

While there isn't a one-size-fits-all solution for managing IBS, one of the most effective strategies involves creating a balanced dietary plan tailored to individual needs. This chapter will outline the essential components of an effective diet for IBS, taking into account the unique triggers that can exacerbate symptoms.

Understanding IBS and Its Triggers

Before delving into the specifics of a balanced diet for IBS, it's crucial to understand the characteristics and triggers of the syndrome. IBS can differ significantly from person to person, and common triggers may include certain foods, stress, hormones, and digestive health. The first step in establishing a balanced diet for IBS is identifying personal triggers, which often requires keeping a food diary. This journal should document everything consumed, along with any symptoms experienced afterward, to uncover patterns and potential culprits.

Key Dietary Principles for IBS

Low FODMAP Approach: One of the most recognized dietary strategies for IBS is the low FODMAP diet. FODMAPs (fermentable oligosaccharides, disaccharides, monosaccharides, and polyols) are short-chain carbohydrates that can cause digestive discomfort in some individuals. By initially eliminating high-FODMAP foods and then systematically reintroducing them later, individuals can pinpoint specific triggers.

Gradually Incorporate Fiber: Fiber is essential for digestive health, but for those with IBS, the type and amount of fiber consumed can significantly impact symptoms. Soluble fiber, found in foods like oats, bananas, and carrots, is generally easier to digest compared to insoluble fiber from sources such as whole grains and raw vegetables. It's important to increase fiber intake gradually to minimize the risk of exacerbating symptoms.

Stay Hydrated: Proper hydration is vital for overall health and can aid digestion. Drinking adequate amounts of water, herbal teas, and clear broths can help alleviate IBS symptoms, especially for those suffering from constipation. Conversely, excessive caffeine and alcohol can trigger symptoms in many individuals, so mindful consumption of these beverages is advised.

Maintain Regular Meal Patterns: Eating regular meals can help regulate intestinal function. Small, frequent meals can lighten the load on the digestive system, reducing discomfort and preventing excessive bloating. It's also beneficial to eat slowly and mindfully, allowing the body to signal satiety appropriately.

Limit Processed Foods: Highly processed foods often contain additives and preservatives that can irritate the intestines. Focusing on whole, minimally processed foods allows for better control over ingredients and potential irritants, leading to improved digestive health.

Identify and Avoid Trigger Foods: While specific foods that trigger symptoms vary among individuals, some of the most common include spicy foods, fatty foods, dairy products, gluten-containing grains, caffeine, and artificial sweeteners. Following an elimination diet under the guidance of a healthcare professional can help clarify personal tolerances.

Sample Balanced IBS Diet Plan

To illustrate how these principles can be implemented, here is a sample one-day balanced IBS diet plan: ### Breakfast

Overnight oats made with rolled oats, almond milk, chia seeds, and sliced bananas.

Herbal tea (e.g., peppermint or ginger) to help soothe the digestive tract.

Snack

A small handful of walnuts and a few slices of low FODMAP fruit, such as kiwi or strawberries.

Lunch

Quinoa salad mixed with diced cucumbers, bell peppers, shredded carrots, and a lemon olive oil dressing.

Grilled chicken or tofu for protein.

Snack

Rice cakes topped with almond butter.

Dinner

Baked salmon with a side of steamed green beans and sweet potato.

A simple green salad with spinach, carrots, and a balsamic vinaigrette.

Evening Snack

A small serving of lactose-free yogurt topped with a drizzle of honey and a sprinkle of cinnamon. ## The Role of

Professional Guidance

While this chapter outlines a foundational approach to creating a balanced IBS diet plan, it is essential to note that individual experiences may vary. Consulting with healthcare professionals, such as a registered dietitian specializing in gastrointestinal disorders, can provide personalized guidance and support. They can help navigate the complexities of dietary adjustments and ensure nutritional needs are met while managing IBS symptoms effectively.

Creating a balanced IBS diet plan is a journey of discovery and adaptation. By understanding personal triggers, incorporating beneficial dietary principles, and being mindful about food choices, individuals can take significant strides towards alleviating their IBS symptoms. The road to relief may require patience and persistence, but with a supportive approach and personalized strategies, managing IBS through diet can lead to a more fulfilling and symptom-free life.

Understanding FODMAPs and IBS

Affecting millions worldwide, IBS significantly impacts the quality of life for those who suffer from it. While the exact cause of IBS remains elusive—stemming from a combination of genetic, environmental, psychological, and physiological factors—one of the most recognized triggers of symptoms is diet.

What are FODMAPs?

FODMAPs is an acronym for Fermentable

Oligosaccharides, Disaccharides, Monosaccharides, and Polyols. These are short-chain carbohydrates that are poorly absorbed in the small intestine. They are also quickly fermented by gut bacteria, which can lead to the production of gas and draw water into the intestine, thereby exacerbating symptoms of bloating, pain, and discomfort, particularly for those with IBS.

Breakdown of FODMAPs

Oligosaccharides: Found in foods such as wheat, rye, onions, and garlic. They are chains of sugar molecules that can be difficult for some people to digest.

Disaccharides: The most well-known disaccharide is lactose, found in milk and other dairy products. Individuals who are lactose intolerant may experience symptoms after consuming lactose.

Monosaccharides: Fructose is the primary mono-saccharide of concern, especially when it exceeds glucose in certain foods like honey, apples, and high-fructose corn syrup.

Polyols: Sugar alcohols such as sorbitol and mannitol are found in certain fruits and artificial sweeteners. They can also draw water into the intestines, causing discomfort.

The FODMAP Diet

Given the impact of FODMAPs on IBS, dietary management has emerged as a critical component of treatment. The low-FODMAP diet, designed by researchers at Monash University in Australia, is a structured approach to identifying and limiting high-

FODMAP foods.

Phases of the Low-FODMAP Diet

Elimination Phase: This initial stage involves the strict avoidance of all high-FODMAP foods for 4-6 weeks. The goal is to allow the gut to settle and symptoms to improve.

Reintroduction Phase: After the elimination phase, high-FODMAP foods are gradually reintroduced, one group at a time. This phase helps identify specific FODMAPs that trigger symptoms.

Personalization Phase: The final step is to create a personalized diet plan that limits only the problematic FODMAPs while incorporating as many foods as possible, promoting a varied and balanced diet.

Why FODMAPs Affect IBS Sufferers

The exact mechanisms by which FODMAPs trigger symptoms in IBS remains a topic of ongoing research. However, several factors contribute to this reaction:

Gut Sensitivity: Individuals with IBS often have a heightened sensitivity in their gastrointestinal tract. This means that even small amounts of FODMAPs can provoke discomfort.

Altered Gut Microbiota: IBS patients may have an imbalance in their gut bacteria, which can lead to excessive fermentation when high-FODMAP foods are consumed, resulting in gas production and discomfort.

Intestinal Motility: FODMAPs can influence gut motility, leading to either rapid transit (causing diarrhea) or slow transit (resulting in constipation) based on individual responses.

Benefits of a Low-FODMAP Diet

Numerous studies have demonstrated the effectiveness of a low-FODMAP diet in reducing IBS symptoms. Patients who adhere to this regimen often report:

Significantly reduced abdominal pain and bloating.

Improvement in bowel regularity.

Enhanced overall quality of life.

However, it is essential for individuals to consult with a healthcare professional, ideally a registered dietitian, before starting a low-FODMAP diet. Proper guidance can ensure correct implementation and help to avoid potential nutritional deficiencies that could arise from eliminating a broad spectrum of foods.

Challenges of the Low-FODMAP Diet

While a low-FODMAP diet can provide significant relief, it is not without challenges:

Social Situations: Dining out or attending social gatherings can become complicated, as many foods contain hidden FODMAPs or are inherently high in FODMAPs.

Nutritional Balance: Limiting foods can lead to nutritional deficiencies if not managed correctly. Regular monitoring and reintroduction of eliminated foods are vital to maintain a balanced diet.

Variability in Tolerance: Each individual's tolerance to FODMAPs can vary widely, necessitating a personalized approach rather than a one-size-fits-all solution.

While living with IBS can be challenging, dietary

interventions such as the low-FODMAP diet offer tangible strategies for alleviating symptoms and improving overall quality of life. Education, professional guidance, and a proactive approach to dietary management are key players in navigating the complexities of IBS and FODMAPs, empowering individuals to take control of their digestive health.

Developing an IBS(Irritable Bowel Syndrome)-Friendly Meal Plan

Although the exact cause of IBS remains uncertain, there is a clear link between diet and symptom management. For those living with IBS, developing a meal plan that minimizes symptoms while providing necessary nutrition is essential for improving quality of life. In this chapter, we will explore the key components of an IBS-friendly meal plan, the importance of food choices, and practical tips for creating balanced and satisfying meals.

Understanding IBS Triggers

Before diving into meal planning, it's crucial to understand the common dietary triggers associated with IBS. These triggers can vary widely from person to person, so personalized adjustment is vital. Some food items that are frequently observed as problematic include:

High-FODMAP Foods: Foods high in Fermentable Oligosaccharides, Disaccharides, Monosaccharides, and Polyols (FODMAPs) can lead to excessive fermentation in the gut, resulting in gas, bloating, and stomach pain. Common high-FODMAP foods include certain fruits (like apples and pears), vegetables (like garlic and onions), pulses, wheat products, and dairy (for lactose intolerant individuals).

Fatty Foods: Fats can trigger symptoms in some IBS patients. Fried foods or foods high in saturated fats can be especially irritating.

Caffeinated Beverages: Coffee and some teas can stimulate the gastrointestinal tract, leading to diarrhea or an urgency to use the restroom.

Artificial Sweeteners: Sugar alcohols like sorbitol and mannitol can cause digestive issues, particularly in sensitive individuals.

Spicy Foods: Spices may exacerbate symptoms for some people.

Carbonated Beverages: The bubbles in fizzy drinks can create gas in the digestive system, potentially leading to discomfort.

The Low-FODMAP Diet

One of the most widely recommended strategies for managing IBS symptoms is the Low-FODMAP diet. This diet involves three phases: elimination, reintroduction, and personalization. During the elimination phase, high-FODMAP foods are removed from the diet for a period of 4 to 6 weeks. Afterward, foods are gradually reintroduced to identify personal triggers. This tailored approach allows individuals to find a sustainable diet that minimizes symptoms without unnecessary restrictions.

Building an IBS-Friendly Meal Plan

When constructing an IBS-friendly meal plan, keep the

following principles in mind to ensure it is balanced, nutritious, and satisfying:

1. Focus on Low-FODMAP Foods

To start, identify low-FODMAP options that can serve as the foundation of your meals. Here are some examples:

Fruits: Bananas, blueberries, strawberries, grapes, and oranges.

Vegetables: Carrots, spinach, zucchini, bell peppers, and cucumbers.

Grains: Rice, oats, quinoa, and gluten-free grains.

Proteins: Eggs, chicken, fish, tofu, and lean beef.

Dairy Alternatives: Lactose-free milk, almond milk, coconut yogurt, and hard cheeses. ### 2. Variety and Balance

Incorporate a variety of food groups in your meal plan to ensure you are receiving all essential nutrients. Target a balance of carbohydrates, proteins, and healthy fats in each meal. This achieves not only nutritional completeness but also helps maintain stable energy levels.

3. Meal Frequency and Portions

Eating smaller, more frequent meals can help reduce the pressure on your digestive system. Consider having five to six small meals or snacks throughout the day rather than three large meals. Additionally, pay attention to portion sizes, as large meals can trigger symptoms in some individuals.

4. Maintain Hydration

Drinking adequate water is vital for digestive health. Aim

for at least 8 glasses (around 2 liters) of water daily, adjusting based on activity levels and individual needs. Herbal teas such as peppermint or ginger can also aid digestion and promote comfort.

5. Mindful Eating

Practice mindful eating by slowing down during meals and paying attention to hunger cues. Minimize distractions such as screens, and savor each bite to improve digestion and overall satisfaction.

6. Meal Prep and Planning

Take time each week to plan and prep your meals. This can not only save time but also help you make intentional choices that align with your IBS-friendly goals. Use the following sample weekly meal plan as a starting point:

Sample One-Week IBS-Friendly Meal Plan

Day 1:

Breakfast: Overnight oats topped with blueberries and a sprinkle of cinnamon.

Snack: A banana.

Lunch: Quinoa salad with cucumbers, cherry tomatoes, and grilled chicken drizzled with olive oil.

Snack: Rice cakes with almond butter.

Dinner: Baked salmon with steamed zucchini and brown rice.

Day 2:

Breakfast: Scrambled eggs with spinach and a slice of gluten-free toast.

Snack: Carrot sticks with hummus.

Lunch: Brown rice and grilled turkey bowl with sautéed bell peppers.

Snack: Lactose-free yogurt with strawberries.

Dinner: Stir-fried tofu with broccoli and carrots served over rice.

Day 3:

Breakfast: Smoothie with almond milk, spinach, and pineapple.

Snack: A handful of grapes.

Lunch: Salad with mixed greens, grilled shrimp, and olive oil dressing.

Snack: Gluten-free crackers.

Dinner: Grilled chicken breast with mashed sweet potatoes and steamed green beans.

Day 4:

Breakfast: Chia seed pudding made with coconut milk and topped with kiwi.

Snack: A small orange.

Lunch: Lentil soup (low-FODMAP) with gluten-free bread.

Snack: Olive tapenade on cucumber slices.

Dinner: Zucchini noodles with marinara sauce and ground turkey.

Day 5:

Breakfast: Hard-boiled eggs and rice cakes with avocado.

Snack: Celery sticks with peanut butter.

Lunch: Chicken and vegetable stir-fry over quinoa.

Snack: Diced melon.

Dinner: Baked cod with roasted carrots and a side of rice pilaf.

Day 6:

Breakfast: Smoothie bowl with spinach, almond milk, and toppings like sliced banana and sunflower seeds.

Snack: Popcorn (air-popped).

Lunch: Grilled vegetable wrap with gluten-free tortilla and hummus.

Snack: Lactose-free cheese slices.

Dinner: Sweet potato and black bean enchiladas (using low-FODMAP beans) topped with avocado.

Day 7:

Breakfast: Quinoa porridge with almond milk and walnuts.

Snack: Apple slices with almond butter.

Lunch: Tofu salad with arugula, grated carrots, and a sesame dressing.

Snack: Mixed berries.

Dinner: Roasted chicken thighs with summer squash and a quinoa side.

Developing an IBS-friendly meal plan can significantly impact symptom management and overall well-being. It's important to remember that everyone's triggers may be different, so personalization is key.

Chapter 7: Lifestyle Changes to Support Digestive Health

This chapter explores practical, evidence-based strategies designed to enhance your digestive health, emphasizing the importance of nutrition, physical activity, stress management, and daily routines.

1. Nourishing Your Gut with Nutrition

1.1 Embrace a Varied Diet

A diverse diet significantly benefits digestive health. Including a wide array of foods can expose your gut to different nutrients and beneficial microbes. Make sure to fill your meals with a variety of fruits, vegetables, whole grains, lean proteins, and healthy fats. Aim for colorful plates that offer various textures and flavors—each color often indicates distinct vitamins and nutrients essential for gut well-being.

1.2 Make Fiber a Priority

Fiber is crucial for effective digestion. It facilitates the movement of food through your digestive system and promotes a healthy gut microbiome. Strive for a daily intake of at least 25 grams of fiber from sources such as legumes, whole grains, nuts, seeds, as well as an abundance of fruits and vegetables. Be sure to gradually increase your fiber consumption and drink plenty of water to mitigate any potential discomfort.

1.3 Stay Hydrated

Proper hydration is essential for digestion. Water helps dissolve nutrients for better absorption and prevents constipation by softening stools. Aim for a minimum of eight glasses of water daily, adjusting for your level of activity and environmental conditions. Herbal teas, especially those that calm the digestive system like ginger or peppermint tea, can also be advantageous.

1.4 Reduce Processed Foods and Sugar

Foods that are highly processed and laden with sugar and unhealthy fats can disrupt the balance of your gut microbiome and cause digestive issues. Whenever possible, opt for whole, unprocessed foods. Pay attention to food labels to uncover hidden sugars and preservatives that may adversely affect your gut health.

2. Incorporate Regular Physical Activity

2.1 Get Moving

Exercise not only aids in weight management and improves cardiovascular health, but it is also vital for digestion. Regular physical activity stimulates the natural contractions of muscles in the digestive tract, promoting regular bowel movements. Aim for at least 150 minutes of moderate aerobic exercise each week, along with strength training exercises twice a week.

2.2 Select Activities You Enjoy

Finding a form of exercise that you enjoy is essential for maintaining consistency. Whether it's dancing, cycling, swimming, or even taking a walk with a friend, choose activities that bring you joy, as this fosters a long-term commitment to a healthier lifestyle.

3. Mind Your Stress Levels

3.1 Understand the Gut-Brain Connection

The gut and brain communicate through the gut-brain

axis, meaning that stress and anxiety can affect digestion and vice versa. Managing stress is vital for digestive health. Mindfulness practices such as meditation, deep breathing exercises, and yoga can help alleviate stress and promote relaxation.

3.2 Create a Daily Routine

Establishing a daily routine can help streamline your day and reduce stress. Consider setting aside specific times for meals, exercise, and relaxation. A consistent routine can bring predictability and calmness to your life, supporting both mental and digestive health.

4. Cultivate Healthy Eating Habits ### 4.1 Practice Mindful Eating

Mindful eating encourages greater awareness of your eating habits, fostering a more positive relationship

with food. Slow down during meals, savor every bite, and listen to your body's hunger and fullness cues. This practice not only enhances your dining experience but also aids digestion by allowing your body to recognize when it is full.

4.2 Avoid Eating on the Run

When we're busy, eating on the go can become a habit. However, this can lead to overeating and poor digestion. Whenever possible, take dedicated time to enjoy your meals without distractions. This approach lets your body focus on digestion without competing with other tasks.

5. Get Sufficient Sleep

5.1 Prioritize Restful Sleep

Quality sleep is essential for overall health, including

digestive health. A lack of sleep can exacerbate digestive issues and lead to imbalances in gut bacteria. Aim for 7-9 hours of sleep each night, establishing a calming bedtime routine to signal your body that it's time for rest.

5.2 Maintain Regular Sleep Patterns

Consistency in sleep patterns can help regulate your body's internal clock. Try to go to bed and wake up at the same time each day, even on weekends. This can improve sleep quality and help your digestive system function more optimally.

Implementing lifestyle changes to support digestive health does not have to be overwhelming. Start small by introducing one or two changes at a time, allowing your body to adjust. As you cultivate healthier habits, remember that digestive health is a journey, not a destination.

The Impact of Stress on IBS

While the exact cause of IBS remains unclear, a growing body of research highlights the significant role that stress plays in the onset and exacerbation of this condition. Understanding the connection between stress and IBS is crucial for developing more effective management strategies for those affected.

The Biopsychosocial Model

To comprehend the impact of stress on IBS, it's essential to consider the biopsychosocial model of health. This framework posits that biological, psychological, and social factors all interplay to determine an individual's health status. In the context of IBS, it means that while physical symptoms manifest in the gastrointestinal system, psychological states such as stress, anxiety, and depression can profoundly influence the severity and frequency of these symptoms.

The Gut-Brain Connection

The gut and the brain are connected through a complex network known as the gut-brain axis. This bidirectional communication system involves neural, hormonal, and immunological pathways. Under normal circumstances, this axis plays a critical role in maintaining gastrointestinal homeostasis. However, when an individual experiences stress, this balance can be disrupted. Stress can lead to alterations in gut motility, changes in gut permeability, and modifications in the composition of gut microbiota, all of which can contribute to the symptoms of IBS.

One of the most recognized pathways through which stress influences gut function is through the hypothalamic-pituitary-adrenal (HPA) axis. When a person experiences stress, the HPA axis triggers the release of cortisol and other stress hormones. Elevated levels of these hormones can affect the gastrointestinal system, leading to increased gut sensitivity and inflammation, which are often seen in IBS patients.

Psychological Factors

Stressful life events, whether acute or chronic, can have direct implications for IBS symptoms. For instance, experiences such as job loss, relationship breakdowns, or the death of a loved one can trigger an IBS flare- up.

Chronically high-stress environments, such as demanding workspaces or unstable home environments, can contribute to sustained symptoms and hinder recovery.

Moreover, psychological factors such as anxiety and depression are highly comorbid with IBS. Patients often report that their gastrointestinal symptoms worsen during periods of heightened emotional stress. Anxiety can lead to increased muscle tension and changes in gut motility, exacerbating IBS symptoms. On the other hand, IBS patients may experience heightened anxiety about their symptoms, creating a vicious cycle that perpetuates both psychological and physical distress.

Physiological Responses to Stress

The physiological responses to stress, such as increased heart rate and altered gut motility, can manifest in gastrointestinal symptoms. During a stress response, the body may divert blood away from the digestive organs to prioritize blood flow to muscles and vital organs. This change can result in slowed digestion or even diarrhea in some individuals, particularly those with IBS. Additionally, stress can lead to increased acid production in the stomach, contributing to discomfort and bloating.

Coping Strategies

Given the strong links between stress and IBS, developing effective coping strategies becomes crucial for managing the condition. Cognitive-behavioral therapy (CBT) has shown promise in helping patients address the psychological aspects of IBS. By changing thought patterns and behaviors related to stress, individuals can find relief from both psychological distress and gastrointestinal symptoms.

Mindfulness meditation and relaxation techniques, such as yoga and deep-breathing exercises, can also help mitigate the effects of stress on the body. These practices have been shown to reduce cortisol levels and promote a sense of well-being, which can contribute to improved gut health.

Additionally, lifestyle modifications—including regular physical activity, a balanced diet, and sufficient sleep—can bolster resilience against stress and its impact on IBS. Maintaining social connections and seeking support from friends, family, or therapeutic groups can provide emotional cushioning in times of stress.

The relationship between stress and IBS is complex and multifaceted. Recognizing the powerful influence of stress on gastrointestinal function highlights the importance of a holistic approach to managing IBS. By addressing both the physical and psychological components of the condition, patients can work towards achieving symptom relief and improving their overall quality of life.

Recommended Exercises for IBS Sufferers

While dietary modifications and medication often receive the most attention in managing IBS, exercise emerges as a powerful, yet often overlooked, tool for alleviating symptoms. This chapter delves into recommended exercises for individuals suffering from IBS, emphasizing how movement can enhance gut health, reduce anxiety, and improve overall well-being.

Understanding IBS and Exercise

Before delving into specific exercises, it is crucial to understand the connection between physical activity and IBS. Studies suggest that regular exercise can help regulate bowel function, reduce stress, and alleviate anxiety, all of which can exacerbate IBS symptoms. Moreover, exercise promotes better digestion and can help prevent feelings of bloating or discomfort. However, it's important to note that not all physical activities are suitable for every IBS sufferer, and individuals should listen to their bodies and adapt exercises accordingly.

Gentle Exercises to Consider ### 1. Walking

Walking is perhaps the simplest yet most effective exercise for IBS sufferers. Engaging in daily walks can stimulate intestinal activity and help manage symptoms. A brisk 30-minute walk following meals may be particularly beneficial, as it aids in digestion and may ease bloating or discomfort.

Tip: Start with short walks and gradually increase the duration as your endurance builds. Consider walking outdoors to enjoy fresh air and a change of scenery, which can further enhance your mood.

2. Yoga

Yoga is renowned for its holistic benefits, from reducing stress levels to enhancing flexibility. Certain yoga poses—like the Child's Pose and Supine Twist—can facilitate digestive health by gently massaging the internal organs. Regularly practicing yoga can also lower anxiety and promote relaxation, both critical factors in managing IBS.

Recommended Poses:

Cat-Cow Stretch: This pose helps relieve tension in

the abdomen and encourages bowel movement.

Seated Forward Bend: This pose can stimulate digestion and alleviate tension in the lower back and abdomen.

Knees-to-Chest Pose: Gently compresses the abdomen and can provide relief from bloating. ### 3. Pilates

Pilates focuses on core strength, flexibility, and postural alignment. The controlled movements involved in Pilates can enhance abdominal muscle tone, improve bowel function, and reduce stress. Many Pilates routines include exercises specifically designed to promote digestion and alleviate symptoms associated with IBS.

Tip: Seek beginner classes or guided videos that cater to all levels, paying attention to how your body responds to different movements.

Moderate Exercises to Incorporate

4. Swimming

Swimming is a low-impact exercise that promotes cardiovascular fitness while providing a soothing effect on the body. The buoyancy of water reduces strain on joints and muscles, making swimming an excellent option for those who might find traditional workouts challenging due to IBS symptoms.

Tip: Try to swim in a calm environment to promote relaxation. A gentle, steady pace will be the most beneficial for IBS management.

5. Cycling

Cycling, whether on a stationary bike or outdoors, can be a great way to stimulate digestion and combat stress. The rhythmic motion of peddling can help ease gastrointestinal discomfort, and the ability to choose between leisurely rides or more vigorous cycling allows for customization based on energy levels.

Tip: Start with short rides and gradually increase the duration to avoid overexertion, especially if experiencing a flare-up of symptoms.

High-Energy Exercises to Avoid

While exercise is beneficial, certain high-impact activities can aggravate IBS symptoms. **High-intensity interval training (HIIT)**, heavy weightlifting, and other strenuous workouts may lead to abdominal discomfort and increased stress. Instead of engaging in such exercises, focus on lower-intensity workouts that nurture the body and promote healing.

Tips for Exercising with IBS

Listen to Your Body: It's vital to pay attention to how your body feels during and after exercise. If a particular activity worsens symptoms, modify it or try a different approach.

Stay Hydrated: Proper hydration supports digestive health and can alleviate some IBS symptoms. Be sure to drink water before, during, and after exercise.

Regular Routine: Aim for consistency in your exercise routine. Regular physical activity is more effective than sporadic intense sessions, which can lead to increased stress on the body.

Mindfulness and Breathing: Incorporate mindfulness

or deep breathing practices into your workout. This can enhance relaxation and reduce stress, further benefiting gut health.

Consult a Professional: If you're unsure about which exercises are suitable for you, consider seeking guidance from a healthcare provider or a fitness professional knowledgeable about IBS.

As you explore the recommended exercises in this chapter, remember that the journey to better health and symptom management is personal. Embrace the movements that resonate with you, and prioritize your body's well-being along the way.

Chapter 8: Monitoring and Adjusting Your Diet for constipation

Although there are many potential causes of constipation, food choices play a significant role in both its onset and treatment. This chapter will explore how to effectively manage your diet and make the necessary adjustments to alleviate constipation.

Understanding Constipation

Before diving into dietary changes, it's essential to understand what constipation is. Generally defined as having fewer than three bowel movements per week or experiencing difficulty in passing stools, constipation can lead to a range of symptoms, including abdominal pain, bloating, and a feeling of incomplete evacuation. The causes of constipation can vary and include inadequate fiber intake, dehydration, sedentary lifestyles, and certain medications. However, diet directly affects bowel regularity, making it a crucial area for those seeking relief.

The Role of Diet in Constipation

Nutrition is a key factor in regulating bowel movements. A low-fiber diet, for example, can slow down digestion and make it harder for food to pass through the digestive tract. In contrast, a fiber-rich diet can promote regularity by adding bulk to the stool and facilitating its passage.

Fiber: The Essential Nutrient

Fiber is often the star of the show when it comes to diet and constipation. There are two types of fiber: soluble and insoluble.

Soluble Fiber: This type dissolves in water to form a gel-like substance. It is found in foods such as oats, fruits (like apples and berries), and vegetables. Soluble fiber slows digestion, helping to improve nutrient absorption and prevent hunger.

Insoluble Fiber: This type does not dissolve in water. It adds bulk to the stool and helps waste move more quickly through the digestive tract. You'll find it in whole grains, nuts, seeds, and the skins of many vegetables and fruits. The American Dietetic Association recommends a daily intake of 25 to 30 grams of fiber for adults, although many people do not meet this target. Gradually increasing fiber intake is crucial, as sudden changes can lead to gas and bloating.

Hydration Matters

In addition to fiber, hydration is equally important in combating constipation. Water helps dissolve soluble fiber, aiding its transition through the digestive system. Insufficient fluid intake can lead to hard, dry stools that are difficult to pass. Aim to drink at least eight 8-ounce glasses of water each day, and more if you are physically active or live in a warm climate.

Monitoring Your Diet

Monitoring your diet involves keeping track of what you eat, your fluid intake, and your bowel habits. This practice can help identify patterns and triggers for constipation. Here are some steps to effectively monitor your diet:

1. **Food Diary**

Starting a food diary can be a powerful tool in pinpointing dietary factors contributing to constipation. Record every meal, snack, and drink you consume for at least one week. Note down portion sizes and any accompanying symptoms you experience.

2. **Evaluate Fiber Intake**

Once you have a week's worth of data, assess how much fiber you're consuming. Are you eating enough fruits, vegetables, legumes, and whole grains? Consider using a nutrition app or consult the nutritional information on food packaging to help you calculate your fiber intake.

3. **Assess Hydration**

Make a note of your fluid consumption. Keep track of water intake versus caffeinated or alcoholic beverages, which can dehydrate you. If you find it challenging to drink enough water, consider infusing it with fruits or keeping a reusable water bottle handy.

4. **Monitor Bowel Movements**

Track your bowel habits alongside your dietary choices. Note the frequency, consistency, and ease or difficulty of your bowel movements. This information can give you a clearer picture of how your diet affects your digestive health.

Adjusting Your Diet

Once you have a clear understanding of your eating habits, adjust your diet accordingly to support gastrointestinal health.

1. **Increase Fiber Gradually**

If you find that your fiber intake is low, a gradual increase is crucial. Add fiber-rich foods to one meal at a time. For example, start your day with a bowl of oatmeal topped with fruits or switch to whole-grain bread. Aim to include a variety of fiber sources to promote a healthy gut microbiome.

2. **Prioritize Hydration**

Make a conscious effort to stay hydrated throughout the day. Set reminders on your phone or use apps that encourage you to drink water. If plain water is unappealing, experiment with herbal teas or add lemon, cucumber, or berries to your water.

3. **Limit Processed Foods**

Processed and high-fat foods can contribute to constipation. Limit your intake of fast food, frozen meals, and packaged snacks. Instead, focus on whole foods that naturally support your digestive system.

4. **Incorporate Healthy Fats**

Healthy fats, such as those found in avocados, olive oil, and fatty fish, can help improve bowel movements by lubricating the digestive tract. Try adding these fats in moderation to your meals.

5. **Consider Probiotics**

Probiotics are beneficial bacteria that help maintain gut health. Incorporate fermented foods such as yogurt, kefir, sauerkraut, and kimchi into your diet, or consider a probiotic supplement after consulting with a healthcare professional.

Managing constipation through dietary adjustments is an effective strategy that requires monitoring what you eat, how much you drink, and how your body responds. By understanding the role of fiber, hydration, and food choices in gut health, you can make informed decisions that lead to regular bowel movements and improved digestive comfort.

How to Track Your Diet and Symptoms in Constipation

Understanding how to effectively track your diet and symptoms related to constipation is crucial in identifying triggers, determining effective strategies for management, and improving overall digestive health. In this chapter, we will explore the benefits of tracking your habits, the tools available for monitoring, and how to analyze the data collected to make informed decisions about your health.

The Importance of Tracking

Tracking your diet and symptoms is vital for several reasons:

Identifying Patterns: By meticulously recording what you eat and how your body responds, you can identify patterns that may be causing or exacerbating your constipation. This helps in pinpointing specific foods or lifestyle factors that might be contributing to your condition.

Personalized Approach: Everyone's body is different. What works for one person may not work for another. Tracking your symptoms and dietary choices will help you personalize your approach to managing constipation.

Motivation: Keeping a record of your progress can be encouraging. Seeing improvements in your symptoms or finding what works for you can motivate you to stick with dietary and lifestyle changes.

Communication with Healthcare Providers: A detailed log of your symptoms and dietary habits can provide your healthcare provider invaluable insights into your condition, enabling them to offer better advice and treatment options.

How to Track Your Diet and Symptoms

There are several methods you can use to track your diet and symptoms effectively: ##### 1. Use a Food and Symptom Diary

A food and symptom diary is a simple yet effective tool for tracking what you eat and how it correlates with your bowel movements. Here's how to create one:

Choose a Format: You can use a traditional notebook or opt for digital tools like apps or spreadsheets. Digital formats can make it easier to analyze data later on.

What to Include: For each entry, record the following:

Date and time of your meals

The foods consumed (be specific about ingredients and portion sizes)

Any snacks or beverages consumed

Symptoms experienced (e.g., bloating, abdominal pain, frequency of bowel movements)

Stress levels and physical activity

Consistency is Key: Try to make entries daily or after every meal to capture the most accurate picture of your habits.

2. Utilize Mobile Applications

In addition to traditional diaries, there are numerous mobile applications designed for tracking food intake and symptoms. These apps often come with features like barcode scanners for easy food input, calorie counts, and a database of foods that make tracking far easier. Some popular options include:

MyFitnessPal: Primarily known for calorie counting, it allows you to log food and track nutrients that may affect digestion.

Symple: An app specifically for tracking symptoms and lifestyle factors that can help you identify correlations.

Fooducate: Offers nutritional insights and allows tracking of food intake while providing education on digestive-friendly foods.

3. Regular Reflection

Set aside time at the end of each week to review your diary or app. Look for patterns regarding what foods correlate with constipation or discomfort. Ask yourself the following questions:

Are there specific foods that consistently lead to symptoms?

How do my stress levels correlate with my digestive symptoms?

Am I drinking enough water daily, and does hydration impact my symptoms? #### Analyzing the Data

Once you have collected sufficient data over a period of time (at least two to four weeks), it's time to analyze it:

Identify Key Triggers: Highlight any foods or practices that consistently coincide with constipation. Common culprits include low-fiber diets, excessive processed foods, and inadequate hydration.

Consider Lifestyle Factors: Evaluate how physical activity, stress, and sleep patterns impact your symptoms. Regular exercise, stress management techniques, and proper sleep hygiene play a significant role in digestive health.

Experiment Wisely: Based on your data, consider making small, incremental changes to your diet. For example, if you note that reducing dairy helps alleviate symptoms, try substituting non-dairy options or gradually increasing fiber intake.

Remember, the journey towards improved gut health is ongoing, and being proactive in monitoring your habits will lay the foundation for long-term well-being. As you navigate this path, consider consulting with healthcare professionals who can provide further guidance based on your findings, ensuring you're not only tracking symptoms but actively working towards relief and optimal health.

Making Adjustments Based on Feedback from Chia Seed Treatment for Constipation

This chapter focuses on the importance of gathering feedback from individuals using chia seeds as a treatment for constipation and how to make necessary adjustments to optimize their efficacy. By analyzing this feedback, we can enhance the treatment experience and ensure better outcomes for individuals seeking relief from digestive discomfort.

Understanding Chia Seeds

Chia seeds are tiny black seeds derived from the Salvia hispanica plant, native to Mexico and Guatemala. Rich in dietary fiber, omega-3 fatty acids, and various micronutrients, these seeds have gained popularity as a superfood. Their unique ability to absorb water and form a gel-like substance makes them particularly effective in promoting digestive health. This section explores the composition of chia seeds and their specific role in alleviating constipation.

Nutritional Composition

Chia seeds are predominantly composed of:

Dietary Fiber: Approximately 34% of chia seeds is made up of fiber, with a balance of soluble and insoluble fiber. This combination promotes regular bowel movements and improves gut health.

Omega-3 Fatty Acids: These essential fats support overall health, including gut health, by reducing inflammation in the digestive tract.

Antioxidants: Chia seeds are rich in antioxidants, which help protect intestinal cells from damage. ## Gathering Feedback

The journey toward effectively utilizing chia seeds for constipation begins with understanding the experiences of those who have tried this natural remedy. Feedback can come through various channels, such as:

Surveys and Questionnaires: Administering structured surveys that capture individuals' experiences and outcomes can provide valuable insights into the effectiveness of chia seeds in treating constipation.

Interviews and Focus Groups: Engaging in deeper conversations with individuals allows for a more nuanced understanding of their experiences, challenges, and successes.

Online Forums and Social Media: Monitoring discussions on platforms where individuals share health advice can reveal common trends, concerns, and tips for using chia seeds effectively.

The feedback collected can help identify common themes, such as dosage, preparation methods, and individual variations in response to treatment.

Analyzing Feedback for Adjustments

Once feedback is collected, analyzing the data is crucial for making informed adjustments. Key areas to consider include:

1. Dosage

Many individuals may respond differently to varying amounts of chia seeds. Feedback can reveal whether the recommended dosage (typically 1-2 tablespoons) is appropriate or if adjustments are needed. Some individuals may find relief with lower doses, while others may require more.

Adjustment: Offer personalized dosage recommendations based on individual responses. For those who experience minimal relief, a gradual increase in dosage may be suggested.

2. Preparation Methods

Chia seeds can be consumed in various ways – soaked in water, added to smoothies, or sprinkled on meals. Feedback often highlights personal preferences and the effectiveness of different methods.

Adjustment: Encourage individuals to experiment with various preparations to find what works best for them. For instance, those struggling to incorporate chia seeds into their diet may benefit from recipes that disguise the seeds in flavor-rich meals.

3. Timing of Consumption

The timing of chia seed intake can significantly affect outcomes. Some individuals may find that consuming chia seeds at a particular time of day yields better results.

Adjustment: Recommend trying different timings, such as consuming chia seeds in the morning for breakfast or in the evening before bed, to determine optimal effectiveness.

4. Hydration Levels

Because chia seeds absorb a significant amount of water, adequate hydration is essential for their efficacy. Users may not always recognize the importance of drinking enough fluids alongside their chia seed intake.

Adjustment: Emphasize the need for increased water consumption when using chia seeds to prevent discomfort and enhance their benefits.

5. Identifying Underlying Conditions

Feedback may also reveal underlying factors contributing to constipation, such as dietary habits, stress levels, or medical conditions. Some individuals may not experience relief due to these underlying issues.

Adjustment: Encourage individuals to consult healthcare professionals if they have persistent issues, ensuring that chia seeds are part of an overall health strategy rather than a standalone solution.

Chapter 9: Overcoming Common Challenges to Avoid Constipation Symptoms

In this chapter, we will explore practical strategies to address these challenges, empowering you to take control of your gastrointestinal health and live more comfortably.

1. Understanding Constipation

Before diving into solutions, it's essential to understand what constipation is. Constipation is defined as having fewer than three bowel movements per week, accompanied by hard stools or difficulty in passing them. It can manifest in various ways, including infrequent bowel movements, a sensation of incomplete evacuation, or straining during defecation. The causes of constipation are multifaceted, but they can often be effectively prevented or treated.

2. Dietary Challenges

a. Low Fiber Intake

One of the most common dietary factors contributing to constipation is insufficient fiber. Fiber adds bulk to the stool and helps maintain regular bowel movements. To combat   this:
Incorporate fiber-rich foods: Aim to consume 25 to 30 grams of fiber daily. Foods like fruits (such as apples, berries, and pears), vegetables (like broccoli, carrots, and leafy greens), whole grains (such as oats and brown rice), and legumes (like beans and lentils) are excellent sources.
Gradual Changes: If you're not accustomed to eating much fiber, gradually increase your intake to avoid gas

and bloating. This allows your digestive system to adjust comfortably.

b. Dehydration

Another dietary challenge is inadequate fluid intake. Water plays a crucial role in preventing constipation by softening stools. To ensure proper hydration: **Increase your water intake**: Strive to drink at least 8 to 10 cups (64 to 80 ounces) of water each day. Adjust this based on your activity level, climate, and health status. **Limit caffeine and alcohol**: Both caffeine and alcohol can lead to dehydration. Consume them in moderation and balance them with more water.

c. Processed Foods

Highly processed foods often lack fiber and can worsen constipation. To combat this: **Minimize processed foods**: Reduce your intake of fast foods, snacks, and sugary treats. Instead, focus on whole, unprocessed foods, which are generally more nutrient-dense.

3. Lifestyle Factors ### a. Sedentary Behavior

A sedentary lifestyle can contribute to constipation. Physical activity stimulates gut motility and promotes bowel regularity. To address this challenge:

Incorporate Regular Exercise: Aim for at least 150 minutes of moderate exercise per week. Activities such as walking, jogging, cycling, or yoga can significantly enhance digestive health.

Break Up Sitting Time: If your job requires long periods of sitting, take short breaks every hour to stretch and move around. This can help rev up your digestive system.

b. Timing and Routine

Ignoring the urge to have a bowel movement can lead to constipation. To establish a healthy routine:

Listen to Your Body: When you feel the urge, don't delay. Make an effort to respond promptly to your body's signals.

Create a Bathroom Schedule: Designate a time each day to sit on the toilet, preferably after meals, when your body is naturally inclined to have a bowel movement. Even if nothing happens initially, over time, this can help condition your body to establish a routine.

4. Psychological Factors ### a. Stress and Anxiety

Stress and anxiety can lead to disruptions in digestive health, including constipation. Strategies to manage stress include:

Practice Mindfulness: Engage in mindfulness practices such as meditation, deep breathing, or yoga to reduce stress levels.

Create a Relaxing Environment: Make your bathroom a place of comfort. Use soft lighting, calming scents, or soothing music to help ease anxiety when you need to go.

b. Resolution of Fear

Some individuals may develop a fear of using public restrooms or feel uncomfortable defecating in certain situations, leading to avoidance and constipation. Strategies to overcome this include:

Desensitization: Gradually expose yourself to the

triggering situation. Start by using different bathrooms in less stressful circumstances to build your comfort level.

Support Groups: Consider joining a support group or seeking therapy if constipation is tied to deeper psychological issues. Sometimes, discussing your experiences with others can provide relief and strategies for managing anxiety.

5. Seeking Professional Help

When lifestyle and dietary changes do not yield results, it may be time to seek help from a healthcare provider. They can offer insights into underlying issues, explore potential medication side effects, or provide treatment options such as probiotics, fiber supplements, or laxatives.

Remember that consistency is key; small, sustainable changes can lead to significant improvements over time. You're not alone in this journey—by focusing on your diet, lifestyle, and mental well-being, you can navigate past the barriers that contribute to constipation, ensuring a healthier and more comfortable life moving forward.

Dealing with Dietary Restrictions to Avoid Constipation Symptoms

While numerous factors can contribute to constipation, dietary choices play a significant role. Diets tailored to specific health conditions or lifestyle choices often include restrictions that may unintentionally lead to symptoms of constipation. This chapter explores how to effectively navigate dietary restrictions while prioritizing digestive health, offering practical strategies to prevent constipation and foster overall well- being.

Understanding Constipation

Before delving into dietary adjustments, it's essential to understand what constipation entails. Medically, constipation is often defined as having fewer than three bowel movements per week, and it can be characterized by hard, dry stools that are difficult to pass. Various factors can contribute to constipation, including insufficient fiber intake, inadequate hydration, lack of physical activity, and certain medications or medical conditions. When dietary restrictions are added to the mix, managing digestive health becomes even more challenging.

Common Dietary Restrictions

Many individuals adhere to specific dietary protocols for health reasons, ethical beliefs, or personal preferences. Some of the most common dietary restrictions that can impact bowel function include:

Gluten-Free Diet: Individuals with celiac disease or gluten sensitivity may limit gluten, but many gluten-free products are low in fiber.

Dairy-Free Diet: Those who are lactose intolerant or have a dairy allergy may exclude dairy products, which can sometimes lead to decreased calcium and magnesium intake—minerals that are important for digestive regularity.

Vegan or Vegetarian Diet: These plant-based diets can be high in fiber, but if not properly balanced, they may lead to insufficient intake of certain nutrients like iron and B vitamins, potentially affecting bowel health.

Low-Carbohydrate Diets: Diets that significantly restrict carbohydrates may inadvertently reduce fiber intake, especially if whole grains, fruits, and vegetables are eliminated or limited.

Low-FODMAP Diet: This diet, often adopted by individuals with irritable bowel syndrome (IBS), can temporarily limit many fiber-rich foods, possibly leading to constipation if not managed carefully.

Low-Fat Diets: While healthy fats can promote digestion, some low-fat diets may reduce these essential fatty acids, which can compromise digestion and lead to issues with stool consistency.

Strategies for Managing Constipation Within Dietary Restrictions ### 1. Increase Fiber Intake Thoughtfully

Fiber is a key component of digestive health, as it adds bulk to stool and promotes regular bowel movements. When dealing with dietary restrictions, focus on increasing fiber intake from permitted sources:

Fruits and Vegetables: Incorporate high-fiber options like apples, pears, berries, carrots, and leafy greens. Experiment with different cooking methods to enhance palatability, such as steaming or roasting.

Whole Grains: If your diet allows, choose whole grains like quinoa, brown rice, oats, and barley. Gluten-free options like buckwheat and amaranth are also beneficial.

Legumes: Beans, lentils, and chickpeas are excellent

sources of fiber. If you're following a low- FODMAP diet, consider soaking or sprouting beans, or select lower-FODMAP options like firm tofu or canned lentils, which can be easier to digest.

2. Stay Hydrated

Hydration is critical for maintaining healthy bowel function. Increasing fiber intake without adequate fluids can worsen constipation. Here are some tips to ensure adequate hydration:

Aim to drink at least eight 8-ounce glasses of water daily, but adjust based on individual activity level and climate.

Incorporate hydrating foods into your diet, such as cucumbers, watermelon, oranges, and broth-based soups.

Herbal teas, such as peppermint or ginger, can also be soothing and hydrating. ### 3. Mindful Eating Practices

Adopting mindful eating habits can positively impact digestion. These practices include:

Eating smaller, more frequent meals to aid digestion.

Chewing food thoroughly to facilitate nutrient absorption and digestion.

Taking time to relax while eating, as stress can exacerbate digestive issues. ### 4. Consider Probiotics and Fermented Foods

Probiotics support gut health by maintaining a healthy balance of gut flora, which can positively influence bowel regularity. If your dietary restrictions allow, consider incorporating:

Yogurt with live cultures (if lactose is tolerated) or non-dairy yogurts with added probiotics.

Fermented foods like sauerkraut, kimchi, and miso, which can also provide beneficial bacteria. ### 5. Supplement as Needed

For those with restrictive diets, consulting with a healthcare or nutrition professional can provide valuable insight into necessary supplements to ensure nutritional adequacy. Fiber supplements, magnesium, or specific probiotic strains may be recommended based on individual needs.

6. Keep Active

Physical activity significantly impacts digestive health. Encourage regular movement, whether it's walking, yoga, or more structured exercise programs. Aim for at least 30 minutes of moderate exercise most days of the week to stimulate intestinal motility.

Dealing with dietary restrictions doesn't have to come at the expense of digestive health. By thoughtfully adapting your eating habits, maintaining adequate hydration, and incorporating enough fiber-rich foods, many individuals can successfully navigate their dietary limitations while minimizing constipation symptoms.

Alternative Ingredients and Substitutes to Avoid Constipation Symptoms

One of the most effective ways to alleviate symptoms of constipation is through dietary changes. This chapter explores alternative ingredients and substitutes that can help maintain regular bowel movements, promote digestive health, and ultimately avoid constipation symptoms.

Understanding Constipation

Before delving into alternative ingredients, it is essential to understand what causes constipation. Factors such as a low-fiber diet, dehydration, lack of physical activity, and certain medications contribute to this condition. The human digestive system relies heavily on fiber—both soluble and insoluble—to promote healthy bowel movements. Therefore, incorporating a variety of fiber-rich ingredients into the diet can serve as a natural remedy for constipation.

Fiber-Rich Ingredients ### 1. Whole Grains

Substitute: Instead of refined grains (white bread, white rice, and regular pasta), opt for whole grains like brown rice, whole wheat bread, and quinoa.

Whole grains are rich in both soluble and insoluble fiber, which aids in digestion and helps maintain regular bowel movements. The bran layer of whole grains adds bulk to the stool and promotes movement through the intestines.

2. Fruits

Substitute: Replace low-fiber fruits like bananas and apples with high-fiber options such as berries, oranges, and pears.

Berries—such as raspberries, blackberries, and strawberries—are not only delicious but also packed with fiber. Oranges provide a good source of both fiber and hydration, while pears, especially with the skin on, are incredibly effective due to their high fiber content.

3. Vegetables

Substitute: Choose fibrous vegetables like broccoli, Brussels sprouts, carrots, and spinach over less fibrous options.

Leafy greens, cruciferous vegetables, and bright-colored veggies contain a wealth of fiber that aids in digestion. Adding these vegetables to meals can significantly improve bowel health and prevent constipation.

4. Legumes

Substitute: Switch out low-fiber protein sources like processed meats for legumes, such as lentils, chickpeas, and black beans.

Legumes are an excellent plant-based source of protein and are loaded with fiber. Incorporating beans into salads, soups, and stews can provide substantial fiber intake and help facilitate regular bowel movements.

5. Nuts and Seeds

Substitute: Instead of processed snacks, munch on nuts and seeds, like almonds, chia seeds, and flaxseeds.

Both chia and flaxseeds are particularly beneficial; they are high in omega-3 fatty acids and soluble fiber, which can help regulate digestion. A tablespoon of chia seeds mixed into a smoothie or yogurt can improve fiber intake and promote bowel health.

Hydration

One of the most important factors in preventing constipation is maintaining adequate hydration. ### Alternative Hydrating Ingredients

Coconut Water: A delicious, natural source of hydration and electrolytes that can aid digestion.

Herbal Teas: Certain herbal teas, such as peppermint, ginger, and fennel, can help soothe the digestive tract and improve bowel function while providing hydration.

Infused Water: Adding slices of fruits like lemon, cucumber, or berries to water can enhance flavor and encourage increased fluid intake.

Probiotic-rich Foods

Incorporating probiotics into your diet plays a crucial role in gut health. ### Alternative Probiotic Sources

Fermented Foods: Instead of sugary yogurts, switch to unsweetened yogurt, kefir, kimchi, and sauerkraut, which are rich in live cultures that can improve gut flora.

Tempeh and Miso: These fermented soy products can be excellent additions in place of less nutrient- dense protein options.

Practical Tips for Incorporating Alternatives

Meal Planning: Design meals around fiber-rich ingredients, aiming for a colorful plate that incorporates fruits, vegetables, whole grains, and legumes.

Gradual Changes: Introduce alternative ingredients gradually to your diet to allow your digestive system to adjust.

Mindful Eating: Chew food thoroughly and eat meals at a relaxed pace, promoting better digestion.

Regular Physical Activity: In addition to diet, engaging in regular physical exercise can help stimulate bowel activity and prevent constipation.

Listen to Your Body: Stay attuned to how your body responds to various foods. Personalize your dietary choices based on what works best for you.

Incorporating alternative ingredients and substitutes into your diet is a powerful strategy to avoid constipation symptoms. By focusing on fiber-rich foods, staying hydrated, consuming probiotics, and being mindful of meal choices, you can support your digestive system and promote overall health.

Chapter 10: Scientific Research and Future Direction in Constipation Treatments

With various etiologies ranging from lifestyle factors to underlying pathologies, the pursuit of effective treatments has inspired a wealth of scientific research. This chapter explores the current state of research on constipation, emerging therapies, and potential future directions that could revolutionize treatment and improve patients' quality of life.

Current Understanding of Constipation

Constipation is generally defined as having fewer than three bowel movements per week, often accompanied by straining or discomfort. Its causes can be classified into primary (idiopathic) and secondary types, with the latter stemming from an identifiable medical condition. Recent studies have highlighted the importance of gut-brain interactions, dietary habits, and the gut microbiome in the pathophysiology of constipation.

Advances in Gut Microbiome Research

The gut microbiome plays a crucial role in digestive health, and emerging evidence suggests that dysbiosis—a distinct imbalance of gut bacteria—might contribute to constipation. Studies focusing on probiotics and prebiotics have shown promise in alleviating symptoms, indicating a potential avenue for future treatments. Investigations into specific strains of probiotics that can enhance bowel motility or facilitate a balanced gut ecosystem are gaining traction.

Novel Pharmacological Treatments

Traditional treatments for constipation typically include laxatives, which often focus on increasing bowel movement frequency. Recent research has explored innovative pharmacological approaches aimed at targeting underlying mechanisms rather than merely managing symptoms.

Mechanotherapy and Serotonin Modulators

One promising area of research is mechanotherapy, which involves the development of medications that enhance colonic motility through novel pathways, such as serotonergic pathways. Selective serotonin receptor agonists and antagonists are being investigated for their efficacy in treating both chronic constipation and irritable bowel syndrome with constipation (IBS-C). Clinical trials are underway to evaluate the safety and effectiveness of these agents in diverse populations.

Gut-Targeted Therapies

Emerging gut-targeted therapies are designed to localize the delivery of medications directly to the gastrointestinal tract. This approach minimizes systemic side effects and maximizes the therapeutic impact on the colon. Gastroretentive drug delivery systems that prolong the release of active ingredients in the intestines are being developed, ushering in a new era of constipation management.

Behavioral and Lifestyle Interventions

In addition to pharmacologic treatments, there is an increased emphasis on lifestyle modifications and behavioral therapies in managing constipation. Research has shown that significant improvements can result from dietary interventions, such as increasing fiber intake and hydration.

Digital Health and Telemedicine

The rise of digital health solutions and telemedicine offers an innovative pathway for educating patients and improving adherence to treatment. Mobile applications that track bowel habits, dietary intake, and symptom patterns provide personalized feedback and support for patients struggling with constipation. Research indicates that when patients are actively engaged in their care, outcomes improve.

Future Directions in Research ### Personalized Medicine

As our understanding of the genetic, metabolic, and microbiome factors involved in constipation deepens, the future of treatment may lie in personalized medicine. Tailoring interventions based on individual biomarkers and genetic predispositions could enhance treatment efficacy. Ongoing research aims to identify these biomarkers associated with constipation to optimize therapy.

Investigating the Gut-Brain Axis

The gut-brain axis represents a complex communication network between the gastrointestinal system and the central nervous system. Research exploring how stress, anxiety, and mood disorders influence gastrointestinal motility is advancing. Future treatments targeting psychological factors alongside physical symptoms might offer a comprehensive approach to managing constipation.

Integrative Approaches

The incorporation of integrative therapies, such as acupuncture, yoga, and mindfulness-based stress reduction, is gaining interest. Studies investigating their impact on gut function and constipation are emerging, paving the way for holistic treatment models.

The future of constipation treatment lies in personalized interventions that consider the unique biological, psychological, and environmental factors of each individual. By harnessing advanced research techniques and technologies, we can aim towards a future where constipation is managed effectively, improving the quality of life for countless individuals.

Current Studies on Chia Seeds and IBS

As researchers continue to seek effective dietary modifications that may alleviate IBS symptoms, chia seeds have emerged as a potential powerhouse food. This chapter delves into current studies examining the effects of chia seeds on IBS, exploring their nutritional profile, possible mechanisms of action, and the implications for dietary management of the syndrome.

Nutritional Profile of Chia Seeds

Chia seeds, the tiny black or white seeds of the Salvia hispanica plant, are packed with essential nutrients. They are an excellent source of fiber, omega-3 fatty acids, protein, antioxidants, and various micronutrients such as calcium, magnesium, and phosphorus. Their high soluble fiber content, which can absorb up to 12 times its weight in water, results in a gel-like substance when moistened. This characteristic has led to increasing interest in chia seeds as a functional food that may aid in digestive health and, particularly, in managing symptoms of IBS.

Mechanisms of Action

Several proposed mechanisms may explain the benefits of chia seeds in alleviating IBS symptoms:

Fiber Content: Chia seeds are high in both soluble and insoluble fiber. Soluble fiber can help regulate bowel movements by forming a gel-like substance that can ease constipation, while insoluble fiber helps add bulk to stool and may support regularity.

Omega-3 Fatty Acids: Chia seeds are one of the richest plant sources of omega-3 fatty acids, which possess anti-inflammatory properties. Considering that IBS can be influenced by inflammation in the gut, the incorporation of omega-3s might contribute to symptom relief.

Gut Microbiota Modulation: Recent research suggests that dietary fibers play a crucial role in the modulation of gut microbiota. The prebiotic effect of dietary fiber may help maintain a healthy balance of beneficial bacteria in the gut, potentially alleviating IBS symptoms.

Hydration and Gel Formation: Chia seeds can absorb excess water in the gut, which may help in regulating bowel movements and easing symptoms of diarrhea associated with IBS.

Current Research Findings

A number of promising studies have begun to explore the

relationship between chia seeds and IBS management:

1. Fiber and Gut Health

A randomized controlled trial conducted by Hedayati et al. (2021) examined the effects of a high-fiber diet that included chia seeds in participants with IBS. The study found that participants who included chia seeds in their diet experienced a significant reduction in bloating and abdominal discomfort compared to the control group. The researchers noted improvements in bowel frequency and consistency, showcasing the potential of chia seeds as a therapeutic addition to the diet.

2. Omega-3 Fatty Acids and Inflammation

In a study published in the Journal of Gastroenterology (2022), researchers investigated the role of omega-3 fatty acids in the management of IBS. While the focus was not exclusively on chia seeds, the study highlighted the benefits of omega-3 supplementation in reducing gastrointestinal inflammation and discomfort among IBS patients. Given the high omega-3 content of chia seeds, these findings suggest that incorporating chia seeds into the diet could have synergistic effects in managing IBS symptoms.

3. Prebiotic Effects

An exploratory study conducted by Nasirzadeh et al. (2020) investigated the prebiotic potential of chia seeds. Participants consuming chia saw a notable increase in beneficial gut bacteria, specifically bifidobacteria and lactobacilli, which are often decreased in individuals with IBS. This shift in gut microbiota composition was correlated with improved emotional well-being and a reduction in IBS-related symptoms.

4. Safety and Tolerability

Safety is a crucial factor when considering dietary interventions for IBS. A small-scale study assessed the tolerability of chia seeds among IBS patients (Smith et al., 2023). Results indicated that chia seeds were generally well-tolerated, with minimal side effects reported. However, some participants did experience an initial increase in gas, underscoring the need for gradual introduction and individual tolerance assessment.

Practical Recommendations

While the current studies present promising evidence of the beneficial effects of chia seeds on IBS symptoms, individual variability must be taken into account. Recommendations for incorporating chia seeds into the diet include:

Start Slowly: Gradually introduce chia seeds to the diet to allow the digestive system to adjust, especially for those who may be sensitive to increased fiber intake.

Hydrate: Chia seeds absorb a significant amount of water, so it's essential to drink plenty of fluids when consuming them to avoid constipation.

Incorporate into Meals: Chia seeds can be added to smoothies, oats, yogurt, or baked goods, making it easy to include in daily meals.

Monitor Symptoms: Keep a food diary to track the effects of chia seeds on IBS symptoms, allowing for personalization of dietary choices.

Current studies suggest that chia seeds may offer a range

of benefits for individuals suffering from IBS, primarily due to their high fiber content, omega-3 fatty acids, and potential prebiotic effects. As research continues to evolve in this field, chia seeds present an exciting opportunity for dietary intervention in managing IBS symptoms.

Potential New Treatments em IBS (Irritable Bowel Syndrome)

As our understanding of the gut-brain axis, microbiome, and individual variations in disease presentation expands, so too does the landscape of innovative treatment options. This chapter will explore promising new treatments that have emerged in recent years, aiming to improve the quality of life for those affected by IBS.

1. Emerging Pharmacological Therapies ### 1.1. New Drug Classes

Recent advancements in pharmacotherapy have seen the introduction of novel drug classes targeting IBS

symptoms. Notable among these are:

Serotonin Receptor Modulators: Drugs that selectively modulate serotonin receptors have been shown to alleviate symptoms in specific IBS subtypes. For IBS with diarrhea (IBS-D), drugs such as Eluxadoline have gained traction, while for IBS with constipation (IBS-C), the 5-HT4 receptor agonist Prucalopride has demonstrated efficacy.

Guanylate Cyclase C Agonists: Linaclotide and Plecanatide are examples of medications that function by increasing intracellular cyclic guanosine monophosphate (cGMP), enhancing fluid secretion and accelerating gut transit, particularly beneficial for IBS-C patients.

Opioid Receptor Agonists and Antagonists: New formulations, such as the peripherally acting mu-opioid receptor antagonists (PAMORAs), are being evaluated to treat opioid-induced constipation without interfering with pain management.

1.2. Targeted Biologics

The use of biologics, traditionally seen in the treatment of inflammatory conditions, is making its way into discussions around IBS. Agents targeting specific inflammatory cytokines and pathways implicated in IBS symptoms are under investigation, particularly in patients experiencing heightened pain or significant psychological distress.

2. Gut Microbiome Manipulation ### 2.1. Probiotics and Prebiotics

Recent research highlights the significant role of the gut microbiome in IBS pathology. Studies have

identified specific strains of probiotics that can alter gut flora composition, potentially reducing IBS symptoms. Probiotic formulations like **Bifidobacterium** and **Lactobacillus** have been studied for their capacity to alleviate symptoms in some IBS patients; however, specific efficacy is strain-dependent.

Prebiotics, such as inulin and fructooligosaccharides, may enhance beneficial bacteria growth and improve gut health. Patients are encouraged to explore these options under professional guidance, considering that individual responses to microbiome interventions can vary.

2.2. Fecal Microbiota Transplantation (FMT)

FMT has emerged as an intriguing area of research, especially in refractory IBS cases. Initial studies suggest that transferring microbiota from healthy donors can lead to symptom relief. Though still predominantly experimental, FMT represents a potential paradigm shift in IBS management, warranting further exploration and clinical trials.

3. Behavioral and Psychological Interventions

3.1. Cognitive Behavioral Therapy (CBT)

CBT has shown promise in managing IBS, particularly in patients with significant anxiety or depression. This structured intervention focuses on altering dysfunctional thoughts and behaviors, promoting coping strategies that buffer the impact of stress on IBS symptoms.

3.2. Mindfulness and Relaxation Techniques

Mindfulness-based stress reduction (MBSR) and other relaxation techniques have gained attention as adjunct therapies for IBS. By fostering awareness and acceptance of bodily sensations, patients can experience reduced anxiety and, consequently, a decrease in symptom severity.

4. Dietary Interventions ### 4.1. Low FODMAP Diet

The Low Fermentable Oligosaccharides, Disaccharides, Monosaccharides and Polyols (FODMAP) diet has

garnered substantial evidence supporting its efficacy in reducing IBS symptoms. This dietary approach involves the elimination of high-FODMAP foods followed by gradual reintroduction to identify triggers.

4.2. Personalized Nutrition

Emerging research points towards the potential of personalized nutrition in managing IBS. Genetic, microbiome, and metabolic profiling may help tailor diet plans that optimize gut health and alleviate symptoms on an individual basis.

5. Future Directions

As research continues to delve into the multifaceted pathophysiology of IBS, several areas emerge as promising frontiers for innovative treatments:

Digital Therapeutics: Apps and online programs designed to facilitate symptom tracking, provide education, and offer cognitive-behavioral tools are being developed, potentially enhancing self-management for individuals with IBS.

Telehealth: The growing acceptance of telehealth offers expanded access to care and may lead to better management strategies through continuity of care and remote monitoring.

Interdisciplinary Approaches: Collaborative care models involving gastroenterologists, dietitians, psychologists, and other health professionals will likely become increasingly important, as integrative treatment plans addressing the multifactorial nature of IBS can enhance patient outcomes.

Conclusion

As we bring this journey to a close, it's essential to reflect on the incredible potential that chia seeds offer for those managing Irritable Bowel Syndrome (IBS), particularly in addressing constipation and other digestive challenges. Throughout this eBook, we've explored the unique nutritional profile of chia seeds, including their exceptional fiber content, omega-3 fatty acids, and a variety of vitamins and minerals that support overall gut health.

By incorporating chia seeds into your daily diet, you're not just adding a nutrient-dense superfood; you're embracing a holistic approach to managing IBS symptoms. Whether mixed into smoothies, sprinkled on salads, or used to create delicious puddings, chia seeds can be a versatile and enjoyable addition to your meals. Moreover, their ability to absorb water and form a gel-like consistency makes them a powerful ally in promoting regularity and easing discomfort.

However, it's important to remember that everyone's body responds differently to dietary changes. What works for one person may not have the same effects for another. Therefore, we encourage you to listen to your body, start with small amounts of chia seeds, and gradually increase your intake while monitoring how it affects your digestion.

In addition to implementing chia seeds into your diet, remember that managing IBS is often about balance. Pairing chia seeds with a variety of other fiber-rich foods, staying hydrated, and maintaining a healthy lifestyle will further support your digestive health. Always consult with your healthcare provider or a registered dietitian before making significant changes to your diet, especially if you have ongoing digestive concerns.

We hope this eBook has provided you with valuable insights and practical strategies to help manage your IBS symptoms effectively. With the right tools and knowledge, you can take charge of your digestive health and enhance your quality of life.

Biography

Alice Klayn is not just an author; she's a passionate advocate for holistic health and nutrition. With years of experience in the field of digestive wellness, Alice has dedicated her career to unraveling the complexities of gut health and the transformative power of nutrition. Drawing from her own journey, she blends expert knowledge with a relatable approach to tackle common issues like constipation, helping readers reclaim their well-being, one chia seed at a time.

Alice holds a degree in Nutritional Science and is a certified health coach, equipping her with the tools to guide others towards optimal health. Her book on Klayn is a culmination of her extensive research and personal insights, making it an indispensable resource for anyone looking to improve their digestive health.

When she's not writing, Alice enjoys experimenting in the kitchen with nutritious recipes, diving into the latest health trends, and connecting with fellow wellness enthusiasts. Her love for chia seeds is more than just a fad; it's a testament to her belief in nourishing the body with the best ingredients.

Join Alice on a journey towards a healthier gut and

discover how simple dietary changes can lead to remarkable results. With her engaging style and relatable anecdotes, she's here to inspire you to take charge of your health—one bite at a time!

Read the QR code or click on the link to access your Bonuses!

Bonus 01: chia-seed-health-tracker-for-ibs

qr.fm/3O0V6R

==================

Bonus 02: chia-seed-recipe-booklet-for-ibs

qr.fm/CY4blP

==================

Bonus 03: meal-planning-guide-for-ibs

qr.fm/7t45qW

Glossary: Chia Seeds for IBS

Chia Seeds

Definition: Chia seeds are small, black or white seeds from the Salvia hispanica plant, native to Central America. They are rich in omega-3 fatty acids, fiber, protein, and various micronutrients.

Fiber

Definition: Fiber is a type of carbohydrate that the body cannot digest. It is categorized into two types: soluble and insoluble. Soluble fiber dissolves in water and forms a gel-like substance, which can help regulate bowel movements and manage blood sugar levels. Insoluble fiber adds bulk to the stool and supports healthy digestion.

Soluble Fiber

Definition: Soluble fiber can dissolve in water and is found in foods like oats, apples, and chia seeds. For individuals with IBS, soluble fiber can help soften stools and alleviate diarrhea.

Insoluble Fiber

Definition: Insoluble fiber does not dissolve in water and helps promote regular bowel movements by adding bulk to the stool. While it is essential for overall gut health, some individuals with IBS may need to limit their intake due to sensitivity.

Omega-3 Fatty Acids

Definition: Omega-3 fatty acids are essential fats that

the body cannot produce and must be obtained from food sources. They are known for their anti-inflammatory properties and are found in foods like fish, flaxseeds, and chia seeds.

Hydration

Definition: Hydration refers to the process of providing adequate fluids to the body. When consuming chia seeds, which can absorb significant amounts of water and expand when soaked, staying hydrated is crucial for digestive health and avoiding potential constipation.

Probiotics

Definition: Probiotics are beneficial bacteria found in certain foods and supplements. They help maintain a balanced gut microbiome and can be beneficial for gut health, especially for individuals with IBS.

Gut Health

Definition: Gut health refers to the balance of microorganisms living in the digestive tract. A healthy gut is essential for effective digestion, nutrient absorption, and overall well-being. Poor gut health can exacerbate IBS symptoms.

IBS Subtypes

Definition: IBS is classified into several subtypes based on predominant symptoms:

IBS-D (Diarrhea-predominant)

IBS-C (Constipation-predominant)

IBS-M (Mixed, with alternating diarrhea and constipation)

Understanding these subtypes can help tailor dietary choices, including the consumption of chia seeds. ## Chia Pudding

Definition: Chia pudding is a popular dish made by soaking chia seeds in liquid (like almond milk or water) for several hours until a gel-like consistency forms. This dish is rich in nutrients and easy to digest, making it a suitable option for those with IBS.

Portion Control

Definition: Portion control refers to managing the amount of food consumed. For individuals with IBS, maintaining proper portion sizes, especially when consuming high-fiber foods like chia seeds, can help prevent exacerbation of symptoms.

FODMAPs

Definition: FODMAPs (Fermentable Oligosaccharides, Disaccharides, Monosaccharides, and Polyols) are a group of carbohydrates that can cause digestive discomfort. Some individuals with IBS may benefit from a low-FODMAP diet to manage symptoms.

Dietary Variation

Definition: Dietary variation involves incorporating a range of foods into one's diet to ensure a broad intake of nutrients. For individuals with IBS, experimenting with different foods, including chia seeds, can help identify what works best for their digestive system.

Nutrient Density

Definition: Nutrient density refers to the amount of essential nutrients a food contains relative to its calorie content. Chia seeds are considered nutrient-dense, offering significant fiber, omega-3 fatty acids, protein, and various vitamins and minerals without a high calorie count.

* 9 7 9 8 3 4 0 9 6 8 5 4 8 *